WITHDRAWN

HAIR LOSS

'A very readable and useful book.'
Nursing Standard

'Both informative and emotionally reassuring.'
Essentials

'Terrific little book.'
TV Times

HAIR LOSS

COPING WITH ALOPECIA AREATA
AND THINNING HAIR

Elizabeth Steel

Thorsons
An Imprint of HarperCollinsPublishers

Thorsons
An Imprint of HarperCollins*Publishers*
77–85 Fulham Palace Road,
Hammersmith, London W6 8JB
1160 Battery Street,
San Francisco, California 94111–1213

First published by Thorsons 1988
This revised edition published 1995
1 3 5 7 9 10 8 6 4 2

A catalogue record for this book
is available from the British Library

ISBN 0-7225-2997-X

Printed in Great Britain by
HarperCollinsManufacturing Glasgow

CONTENTS

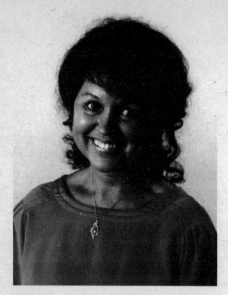

Elizabeth Steel writes from bitter experience. She lost her hair through scalp disease and found that she was not alone . . . that it was happening to thousands of others.

She founded Hairline International, The Alopecia Patients' Society, as a self-help network for those who have lost — or are losing — their hair.

After eight years in wigs and headscarves, her hair grew back. Other alopecia sufferers, she says, can be equally fortunate.

Elizabeth Steel is the pen name of Wendy Jones, the former Midlands TV presenter and producer.

FOREWORD

A lay organization for alopecia sufferers has long been needed in view of the general ignorance surrounding many types of hair loss – a field in which anxiety and fear can be profound and in which many pseudo-scientific experts abound, often with little more than financial motives.

Elizabeth Steel deserves enormous credit for attempting to fill this medical void. She has solicited advice from a great array of medical and scientific experts and listened with the utmost patience and understanding to the problems of hundreds of sufferers. One hopes that this succinct book will in some way be a help to the very many individuals who suffer from alopecia.

Dr Rodney Dawber, MA, MB, Ch.B., FRCP
Consultant dermatologist, John Radcliffe Hospital and clinical lecturer, Oxford

Loss of hair can cause profound emotional difficulties. I have long felt that such a patient society would help sufferers of hair-growth disorders, particularly alopecia areata.

Dr Andrew G Messenger, MD, MB, B.Sc, MRCP
Consultant dermatologist, Royal Hallamshire Hospital, Sheffield

There can be few more distressing situations in life than finding that you are suddenly losing your hair. To discover there is little by way of effective treatment and that the ultimate prognosis depends more on fate than medical intervention is enough to make even the most resilient of characters somewhat despondent.

In such situations the support of others who have been down the same road and the availability of a ready supply of information on current treatments and research is an essential support service. Hairline is therefore a long overdue concept and one which will, I am sure, have the enthusiastic support of doctors and alopecia sufferers.

Dr John D Wilkinson, MB, MRCP
Consultant dermatologist, Wycombe General Hospital, High Wycombe

ACKNOWLEDGEMENT

This book could not have been written without the support and guidance of many doctors. I hope they will accept that some criticisms apply not to the individual specialist so much as to the system and I thank them for all they have done to make this book possible.

INTRODUCTION

When it happened . . .

- Anna, 24, a beautiful nurse, called off her wedding.
- Ross, 45, a former army officer, felt he would never satisfy a woman again.
- Hilary, 35, the sophisticated wife of a city industrialist, spent a fortune trying to get her hair back – only to lose it all in the shower of her Mediterranean villa.
- Joanne, 7, suddenly stopped wearing dresses. She felt like a boy.
- Sally, 18, tried to kill herself with an overdose of alcohol and drugs.
- Duncan Goodhew, swimmer, turned his affliction to advantage. The Olympic gold medallist says, 'If it hadn't happened to me when I was 10 years old I might never have made it as a champion in sport. Adversity either makes or breaks.'

These people have one thing in common. They have lost all their hair, rapidly and frighteningly, through the scalp disease alopecia areata. It can happen to anyone, man or woman, at any age. It happened to me, when I was in my thirties and appearing on television for a living.

It could happen to you.

So you have suddenly lost your hair. Maybe you are only starting to get small bald patches, or perhaps you have lost it all. You are shocked, horrified and panic-stricken.

Of course you are. One minute you are taking your hair for granted – complaining, perhaps, that it is too dry, too greasy or that your hairdresser has cut it too short. Or maybe you just dislike the style. Then *wham!* Out of the blue, for no reason you know of, your hair falls out. The process may take six months or just a day or two. It can even happen overnight.

The result is the same. A scalp made unsightly by large bare patches, a thin top layer of hair you can see through . . . or a shiny, completely bald head. Miserable enough for a man. A downright catastrophe for a woman.

When you suddenly lose your hair as an adult, you feel immediately humiliated. It destroys your confidence in yourself in every aspect of your life.

You see a different person in the mirror. That unfamiliar hairless head – is that mine?

You feel unattractive – how could anyone possibly fancy such a poor, bald freak? To be attractive you need to feel – at least a little – enamoured of yourself. When your hair goes and self-esteem with it, your self-image is shattered.

So, probably, is your sex life. Without hair, many people find that their first problem is sex. Their second problem is sex. And their third problem is sex. To survive severe hair loss you need a whole new outlook on yourself and your relationships.

This book will do more than tell the story of the thousands who suffer. It will also tell you how to survive, how to come out of the situation looking as good as you did before — perhaps even better!

One in a hundred

As many as one in a hundred people lose their hair through the scalp disease alopecia areata, according to leading American dermatologist Dr Sigfrid A. Muller of the Mayo Clinic.

For years, no one has known how many people suffer this freak hair loss. This is because only a tiny percentage of victims ever goes to a hospital. Many don't even see their family doctor. Medical statistics, therefore, reflect only a tiny fraction of the problem.

To find out the true incidence, Dr Muller led a team of doctors in a major epidemiological survey in Rochester, Minnesota, USA. He asked: 'Just how many of the population get this disease?' His conclusion was staggering. Over the next 60 years, he discovered, approximately one per cent of the population will have alopecia areata — not the gentle, gradual balding of old age, but sudden, devastating hair loss which can happen at any time.

Dr Muller emphasizes the good news. He told me that as many as 95 per cent of these cases may be only mild ones, but his earlier research suggests that the number of people who lose *all* their hair could be as high as 30 per cent.

Alopecia areata (from the Greek for 'mangy fox') usually starts with a tiny bald patch the size of a 10 pence piece. Sometimes it becomes diffuse alopecia, spread over the entire scalp. Younger patients often find their alopecia areata begins as a diffuse loss.

When it happened to me, it was first diagnosed as post partum telogen effluvium – hair loss related to a recent pregnancy; later, by a consultant dermatologist, as classic alopecia areata; and later still, by another consultant, as diffuse alopecia.

Worldwide, experts have suspected for the past 30 years that there has been an increase in diffuse alopecia, particularly among women. As far back as 1960, a team of German dermatologists reported an increase in diffuse hair loss in women.[1] This came at a time when – coincidentally – women were beginning to take the contraceptive pill. All over the world, women were swallowing high quantities of the synthetic hormone progestogen.

Several years later, dermatologist Dr Frank E. Cormia of Cornell University, New York, linked cases of female hair loss directly with the pill and suggested that it could trigger 'male pattern' baldness in women, telogen effluvium and other types of diffuse hair loss.[2] His report prompted the question: Is a generation of balding women the price we pay for the convenient chemical?

Alopecia areata is the mystery scalp disease which strikes savagely without warning, so that someone who has had a perfectly normal head of hair suddenly loses it. Hair comes out from the roots in ugly clumps. You may be lucky and have only a small patch, which clears up and never reappears. You may be unlucky and lose the lot – all scalp hair plus eyelashes and eyebrows (alopecia totalis). You may lose all body hair, including scalp (alopecia universalis). Or you may be plagued by odd patches all your life.

At the same time, nails often become pitted and ridged. You won't know why, neither will your doctors. They know the mechanism, that it is almost certainly an auto-immune disease in which some of the white blood cells – the lymphocytes – overwork and produce antibodies which attack the hair follicles as though they were foreign bodies. But doctors don't know what triggers it or, more important, how to stop it.

After years of research across the world, dermatologists admit that they are still baffled. Too often they are forced to tell patients: 'There is nothing we can do. Go home. Learn to live with it.' Or without it! Doctors daily carry out miraculous treatments on tragic cases of cancer, heart disease, polio, but when it comes to the apparently simple fact of baldness there is – too often – little they can do.

When it happened to me, I was perfectly happy with a young family and an exacting career as a television journalist. I felt totally alone and a complete freak. I thought I was the only young woman in the world to go bald, but an article I wrote in a top women's magazine, *Good Housekeeping*, and my radio feature on BBC Radio Four's *Woman's Hour* convinced me I was wrong.

Countless letters poured in, all from people in the same boat. Sudden baldness had isolated them, had caused marital, social and psychological problems. One woman, who had been a glamorous nightclub dancer, confessed: 'There's never a week when I don't consider suicide.' They wrote from the United Kingdom, Europe, America, the Far East . . . All over the world women were spending their lives in headscarves or wigs, terrified of revealing their secret, that underneath they looked like plucked chickens or victims of Chernobyl. Men wrote that alopecia areata (AA) had shattered their confidence and wrecked their relationships. The moth-eaten patches had played havoc with their appearance and made them look slovenly. They felt odd, different from other men.

For years, the subject had been swept under the carpet.

Premature baldness, particularly in a woman, is by no means a seductive sight.

Some doctors, embarrassed perhaps by their inability to help, have blamed it vaguely on stress or shock, or prescribed tranquillizers with advice to 'stop worrying'. Some have suggested that it is imaginary. In a few rare cases, they are right. The patient may have a distorted body image (dysmorphophobia – see page 173). But for most of us, when hair falls out suddenly it is an all too horrifying *fact*.

What kind of hair loss is it?

Generally, we are talking about loss of hair above the normal hair fall of 70 to 140 hairs a day. We all lose this much, probably without noticing.

During its growth – its *anagen* – phase, hair grows approximately half an inch a month. This phase lasts up to six years with a short resting – *telogen* – phase of about three months, when the hair is shed. Normally, about 85 per cent of your hair is in anagen and 15 per cent in telogen.

- **Telogen effluvium** Sometimes hair enters its telogen phase too early. This often happens after childbirth and usually clears up within a few months. In some cases it lasts much longer. The resultant thinning occurs as a kind of 'human moult' and can also happen as the result of a sudden shock – either emotional or physical. It can also happen after a high fever or major surgery.
- **Alopecia androgenetica** This occurs in 95 per cent of men and 50 per cent of women as they grow older. In a few cases, often as a family trait, it happens in younger people. In a man it appears as the familiar receding temples and thin crown of 'male pattern baldness'. In a woman it

usually appears as a diffuse thinning throughout the scalp. It is caused by three factors: age, heredity and the action of androgens (male hormones) on the hair follicles. The commonly used term 'male pattern baldness' can be offensive to women with this problem, as they are unlikely to have any other male characteristics. They are usually completely feminine in every other way! For this reason it is often referred to as 'female pattern baldness' when it occurs in a woman.

The diffuse thinning results in the embarrassment of 'see-through' hair where the scalp is clearly visible through a layer of very sparse hair. As well as happening as women grow older, it also occurs in younger women. Thirteen per cent of pre-menopausal women suffer diffuse loss, as do 37 per cent of women who are post-menopausal. Thinning hair can be just as distressing as to lose hair in actual bald patches. Younger women are sometimes helped by anti-androgen therapy (see page 181).

- **Hereditary/congenital alopecia** This is passed down in families in rare syndromes.
- **Traction alopecia** This is caused by tightly pulled pony tails, braids and chignons. The styles themselves are not to blame but too much pulling and tension does the damage. This is common among West Indians, who love tight braids. Rollers pulled too tightly can also cause it.
- **Friction alopecia** This occurs when hair bands, wigs or hats are too tight. The hair often breaks off.
- **Scarring/Cicatricial alopecia** This is where hair is damaged through an accident and skin/hair follicles suffer permanently, possibly through burns. If the hair follicle is destroyed, there is no hope of re-growth.
- **Hair lost through medical treatment** The drugs

used in chemotherapy treatment for cancer often cause loss of hair. In most cases this returns after the course of chemotherapy and patients need only support and help in choosing wigs for a short period. Western hospitals at first assumed, wrongly, that hair loss would be unimportant to a woman who had come through the experience of cancer. But health professionals now understand the psychological effects of hair loss particularly on a woman patient. When I spoke on hair loss at a recent conference at Addenbrookes Hospital, Cambridge, I was told: 'It is one of the most distressing aspects. Patients always want to know whether they will lose their hair.' Cancer patients now have advice on this aspect as soon as their chemotherapy is discussed – and wig specialists are invited into hospitals to advise patients immediately.

- **Alopecia areata** This is a disease of the scalp in which baldness is patchy and can progress into the loss of all scalp hair (alopecia totalis) or all body hair, including the scalp (alopecia universalis).

Alopecia areata is bewildering and eccentric. Many people report that specialists are unable to help, offering neither counselling nor treatment. Often, when treatments are given, the hair falls out again when they stop.

Faced with this pessimistic situation, it is hardly surprising that some skin specialists behave brusquely to their alopecia patients, retreating behind a mask of 'I am the expert, the qualified doctor,' refusing to explain the condition to them, trotting out soothing banalities: 'It is bound to grow back.' 'Don't worry.' 'You can buy some lovely wigs.' Doctors, after all, are human. Faced with a choice of treatments which rarely work, for a condition they don't fully understand, most human beings could be forgiven for feeling threatened and inadequate – which, I am sure, is how many dermatologists feel.

Can medical advances help?

Doctors know how to suppress the immune system to prevent it from rejecting transplanted organs such as hearts and kidneys. Could those immuno-suppressive drugs be used to prevent the immune system from rejecting the hair as foreign?

Yes, in theory, say dermatologists, but in practice they doubt the advisability of prescribing them to be taken by mouth, as any interference with the immune system might lower resistance to infection. The patient could become very ill. One of this drug group, azathioprine, is occasionally given orally when other treatments have failed but it needs to be carefully monitored.

To play safe and cut out risks, one of the immuno-suppressive drugs, cyclosporine, is currently being tried in a 10 per cent gel to be used topically i.e. applied to the scalp. So far there have been no side-effects on blood pressure or kidneys, but the results of recent trials have been disappointing.

A more recent hope has been the discovery that minoxidil, a drug used to treat high blood pressure, will sometimes encourage hair growth in people with patchy – mild – alopecia (see Chapter 7). This treatment is now marketed in the UK over the pharmacist's counter as Regaine. It has a two per cent solution of minoxidil.

And hope for those who have had severe hair loss for many years seems to lie with the sensitizer diphencyprone, which has actually triggered hair growth in a patient who had been completely bald for 54 years!

The majority of patients, however, receive little medical help. You may see your GP. If the case is severe, he or she may refer you to a consultant dermatologist. But patients are often disappointed. They have received this kind of advice from specialists:

- 'Don't think about yourself so much!'
- 'It might grow back. It might not.'
- To a young wife of 32, who had lost *all* her hair, including eyebrows and eyelashes: 'You can get some very pretty hats these days!'

Hard enough to take when you are grown up, but worse for a child.

- Peppi, 13, slashed her arms with a knife in the playground of her comprehensive school. Her scalp hair had nearly all fallen out and other children were playing games trying to knock her wig off.
- Joanne, aged 9, refused to wear party dresses after she lost all her hair two years ago. 'She suddenly refused to wear anything but shorts and T-shirts,' says her mother. 'She changed from a pretty little girl who loved parties and frills and black patent shoes, to a tomboy.'
- The parents of Laura, aged 13, were stunned by the behaviour of a consultant. Says her father: 'He glanced cursorily at her head and remarked "You're going to have to wear a wig, aren't you?"' Her mother, herself a hospital worker, was equally upset. 'We were given no medication or advice as to how a formerly attractive girl of 13 should be helped to cope with baldness. Laura has twice been suicidal.'

It is perhaps understandable that alopecia areata apparently merits such low priority in hospitals. After all, it neither cripples nor kills. Dermatology is a tiny speciality with fewer than 250 consultants in the UK and 6,000 in the USA. The bad news is that many of them send their patients home with little positive help. Indeed, they often adopt a deliberate policy of inactivity, on the grounds that it is pointless to use uncomfortable, perhaps expensive treatments which may not work.

The good news is that a small group of dedicated dermatologists is seriously involved in research and treatment for alopecia victims. They try very hard to help the patient through the trauma of hair loss.

Dr Andrew Messenger, consultant dermatologist at Sheffield's Royal Hallamshire Hospital, says: 'I see my role here as more than merely to administer treatments. I am here – I hope – to talk with the patient and try to help her through. I try to make time to do this. The dilemma with so many of the treatments we have available is the fact that we have a condition which is in no way physically harmful. But we could cause physical damage with treatments in a case where the original problem is merely cosmetic.'

Some treatments carry a risk. There can be side-effects, such as weight gain, with long-term systemic steroids. Some sensitizers have been found to be mutagenic, i.e. they can change the structure of cells.

Says Dr Messenger: 'It is depressing to treat alopecia. I find it sad that there is so little I can do. I feel sorry for the single people who lose their hair at a time when their looks are crucial – when they are just beginning to make relationships.' The sociological and psychological effects of alopecia are often very serious. Marriages break up; careers are ruined.

The Hairline survival plan

Because so many sufferers wrote to me of their desperation I began to meet them and eventually founded Hairline International – the Alopecia Patients' Society. It is the only alopecia patients' support network in the U.K. and now has members in 20 countries around the world.

Between us, we worked out a survival plan. We may have to live with the condition but there are ways of coping, so that you can even look – and feel – better than you ever did before. There are even advantages in being bald.

You don't believe me? My survival plan is part of this book, to help you through every stage of this illness, with all the day-to-day problems. For too long we have all tried to hide it. We have been inexplicably ashamed and humiliated. We have been terrified that people would laugh at us. But at last we are coming out of the closet and talking openly about our baldness.

Only good can come of it.

PART I

Why?

1

WHEN I LOST MY HAIR

'I felt such a freak . . . when it happened to me.'

I know now, since so many people have been in touch, that I haven't suffered nearly as much as some, particularly the children. I know now that it's 'only hair', after all. To lose it is by no means the end of the world, but at the time you just don't know what's hit you. If this is the way you are feeling at this moment my story may help.

The hairdresser prodded my hair and poked at the wet strands with a tail comb. She said, 'I think you ought to see a doctor. Just to put your mind at rest.'

So it began, my nightmare. On a May morning when the sun beamed on the suburbs and my 15-month-old daughter toddled with a teddy bear beside the basins.

Don't be ridiculous. Only men go bald, or very old ladies in geriatric hospitals. Not me, a young woman – well, comparatively young – with a hectic career as a freelance writer and television journalist.

'Not the career boost I need,' I thought grimly.

My hair was long, dark and one of my greatest assets. 'Damn it all,' I thought crossly, 'I've spent a fortune on it, over the years.' I was always at the hairdresser's. Everyone said so. My family used to joke that if I ever went missing, that was the place to find me. Hair had always been important. In my career, in television, I had a legitimate reason to keep it looking good, though it was doubtful whether my appearances on screen justified the time and money I had squandered all my life on shampoos, sets, tints and blow waves.

Hair had become more than a vanity, almost an obsession. Faithfully, I had followed fashion, back-combed and permed it – even on impulse bleached the whole lot blonde. I could have understood if my hair had fallen out then, but it had hung on happily through all that, amazingly good-tempered.

My bookcase was a shrine to it. Family photographs depicted the results of my many years under the drier. The hair starred, long, dark and shining in all of them. Formal, expertly waved, it fell on to bare brown shoulders above an evening dress. Dramatically, it was swept back under a wide-brimmed hat at the church fête. Shamelessly, it tried to outshine the bride at my best friend's wedding, its ringlets cascading *Pride and Prejudice*-style on to the pink tulle of my bridesmaid's dress.

'You'll laugh about this one day,' I told myself, as the hairdresser busied herself with rollers and pins. 'You'll look back on this as the day you thought you were going bald. How silly!'

But *I was*. Within weeks I had lost all my hair, save for a little tuft hanging on valiantly at the back. Hair fell out steadily, heavily, on my pillow and dressing table, in the shower, on the floor – everywhere. In a shop's fitting room, I pulled off a dress and a great clump of hair with it. Suddenly I saw my bare scalp in the mirror. Shiny, gleaming under the spotlight, it was the stark rounded shape of the Loch Ness monster's head.

'Alopecia areata', diagnosed my family doctor. Such a pretty name. Its name was the only pretty thing about it.

'Probably telogen effluvium', he added, 'post partum alopecia, excessive hair fall after having a baby.'

I had expected the medical profession to know immediately what to do, to hand out a prescription and offer treatment, as they had speedily dealt with all my ailments over the years. That was my first discovery.

FACT: Doctors Know Neither Cause Nor Cure.

'But I'm working next week,' I wailed at my GP. 'I can't appear on television looking like this!' The small patches had spread purposefully. Indoors and out, I covered my nearly bald head with a scarf. The doctor smiled, wry humour shielding him, as always, from the messy humanity paraded daily in his surgery. 'Try your make-up department,' he suggested.

But magic wands are not part of the standard equipment carried by TV make-up departments. Magic – or a miracle – was the only thing which would have made my hair sprout back where once it had grown. Angled bathroom mirrors confirmed that my hair had mostly vanished – totally at the front, over the crown and leaving only that tuft in the nape of my neck.

For a few weeks my skilful hairdresser managed to spread the section at the back enough to cover the front! 'My Arthur Scargill style', I called it. This strange condition had given me a new sympathy for the coal miners' leader and all the politicians who struggle daily to disguise their bald pates in public.

I might just get away with it, I hoped, but the weather was against me! The wind blew on the day I was to appear again in a television show. In the 30 seconds it took me to cross the road to the studios, my hairdresser's painstaking arrangement was destroyed. The studio monitor told me what I already knew – that those pathetic little hairs, no matter how carefully arranged, couldn't possibly hide the bare scalp underneath.

It was hopeless. I tried to compose a letter to the television company but found it impossible. How did I explain? 'I am afraid I have lost all my hair.' It sounded so funny and begged the response: 'How very careless of you.' I visualized the office staff, passing my letter around, secretaries hiding it behind their word processors. 'I know we shouldn't laugh, but have you heard . . ?' The smothered guffaws, the guilty little giggles . . .

FACT: Baldness is Funny – to Everyone Else!
There are so many easy phrases which come as a natural part of the language.

- 'Keep your hair on!'
- 'Tearing your hair out!'
- 'They're driving me hairless!'

I would just have to learn to take it, smile bravely at laboured cracks about Kojak and Yul Brynner.

Friends tried to cheer me with sad little jokes. 'See you at the party,' said my girl friend, after I had told her about it on the phone. 'I expect you'll be the one in the hat!' 'You'll look like a punk rocker,' predicted a cousin.

A late-night TV programme was enjoying a good laugh on the subject. 'Does baldness really matter?' hooted the girl reporter, her own hair thickly fringed and plentiful. She was right. Baldness *is* a joke, if it is just the predictable, slow loss a man usually gets. Receding temples and disappearing crown – first sign of old age, a rueful smile from him and a gentle joke from his wife! But when baldness happens in the space of a week – or even a day or two – to a young man or woman who is instantly an 'oddity' or, even worse, to a child, that's not much of a joke at all.

My husband tried to be kind. 'It will probably do it the world of good in the end,' he observed. Poor man, kind and optimistic by nature. What could he say, faced with the messy tears and rapidly balding head of his once presentable bride?

I struggled with it daily at the dressing table, in a bedroom full of hair. It was everywhere, except on my head!

The family holiday in Majorca was a disaster. Daily I rose at 5 a.m. to battle with heated rollers and the few remaining strands of hair, but travelling in the family's holiday Mini soon blew it away. My father had hired the car to take us around the island. He was downcast when I refused to get out to see the view from the top of a hill. I had seen other tourists clambering out of cars and the women's hair streaming in the wind!

Every evening I took ages with my 'hair' while the family downstairs grew impatient, waiting for me. Silly vain woman, trying to look normal and disguise the head which looked more like a boiled egg every day. 'Don't cry,' said my husband, as tears of self-pity flowed in the hot bedroom, on to the debris of hair lacquer, combs and rollers. 'When we get back you'll go straight to the best specialist we can find, no matter how much it costs.'

He was well meaning, but mistaken.

FACT: No Specialist can Guarantee to Make Hair Grow Again.
Over the years the dermatologists have tried many different techniques, from ultraviolet light to steroids, but the chances of success with any of these treatments is extremely limited. In any case, as the hair often grows back of its own accord,

any apparent success is difficult to evaluate.

Back home, my GP referred me to a consultant dermatologist. He predicted that my hair would probably grow back 'in no time'. 'But you need to get your confidence back,' he said. Shrewd of him to notice that I, who had always been so full of confidence – at least outwardly – had lost it with my hair. Self-regard had slipped away in those frightening few weeks. I felt diminished.

'I'll give you a prescription to get some financial help with wigs,' he added. The situation took on its nightmare quality again. I dreamed last night that I lost all my hair and a doctor was prescribing wigs. Had it really come to that? 'I don't know how you've managed without a wig for so long,' he remarked.

I was still full of questions. Why should I – young, healthy and female – suddenly lose my hair? The sixty-four thousand dollar question remained unanswered. The consultant was frank. 'Let's be honest. We don't know. It could happen to anyone. I could wake up tomorrow with no hair' – a thought he clearly found unlikely.

My GP had suggested that it might have been brought on by childbirth – a theory the consultant dismissed swiftly. 'What? Fifteen months later? Any hair loss connected with birth would have cleared up again in two or three months.' He shook his head, his eyes resting irritably on my daughter, who was rattling the car keys I had given her as a distraction.

'You have a classic case of alopecia areata. The Americans reckon it's all caused by stress.' He grinned. 'But then, they blame stress for everything.'

I was beginning to get the impression that it was some kind of mental crack-up but that no one liked to tell me. 'Are you saying it's a nervous breakdown or something?'

'No. As far as we know, this is an auto-immune disease. The lymphocytes, which are part of the body's defence mechanism and reject anything foreign, overwork and reject the hair follicles. But we don't know what triggers it. We can only surmise that it is worry, anxiety, stress. These days, though, that idea is a bit out of fashion.'

FACT: Doctors Who Once Blamed Stress Now Question This Theory.

The dermatologist was looking at my scalp. 'Have you noticed these tiny white hairs growing in some of the patches, like soft down?' I confessed, 'That's probably my hair's true colour now. I've been tinting it for years.' He disagreed. 'It wouldn't be as white as this, not at your age. It's part of the condition. The hair grows back without pigmentation.' Hair turning white overnight! Hair dropping out! It wasn't real, more like a Victorian melodrama.

He could offer no treatment, only basic blood tests and a health-service contribution towards wigs. I must return to the hospital for these.

Black city centre, stormy July cloudbursts over the hospital, rain saturating me and the baby as I hastened the push-chair into the gloomy grey entrance. I queued with a restless child in the skin clinic. I waited for the blood tests which, according to my consultant, would almost certainly eliminate thyroid deficiency or anaemia as the cause. Then I trekked round bare-bricked corridors to find the department labelled 'Appliances'.

It was empty. Tentatively, I approached two girl typists and asked for the appliance officer. To my surprise, they laughed. I wondered why. Did they think I meant some kind of sexual appliance? Sobering, they offered advice. 'You'll just have to wait. She's probably on the wards.'

I sat down, heavy with the burden of being a nuisance. Soon the baby would be hungry for her tea. Dismally, I decided I should think myself lucky I wasn't queuing up for a wooden leg.

If I had been in need of an artificial limb the appliance officer would probably have been more sympathetic. Eventually, she stomped in, stout and scathing. I had no right, said her narrowing eyes, to be taking up a consultant's time with such trivia.

'Date of birth,' she barked across the office, then repeated the figures at a similar pitch. 'And you want a wig?' Her voice was loud enough to reach every corner of the hospital.

Humble before her, I was silent. 'Right, all you people out there,' I thought savagely. 'Now you know. I'm not only very *old*, I'm bald as well.'

She flourished a form. '£90, please.' I flinched. I had assumed I was getting wigs on the National Health Service and it hadn't occurred to me to bring a cheque book. The appliance officer thought I was objecting to the amount. 'It's only a small contribution towards the real cost,' she pointed out. 'A genuine hair wig would cost you over £200 if you were paying the full price.'

I started to ransack my purse, then stopped. 'I don't have to have two wigs, though. Can't I just take one?'

Her patience, clearly, had worn thin, in years of coping with an ungrateful public. 'I suppose you could, but what will you do when it wants cleaning?'

'Well, the doctor says my own hair will soon grow again.' She didn't say 'Hah', but she thought it, I could tell. She had presumably heard such nonsense before. My optimism must have appeared pathetic. With a swift stroke of her pen, she brought the conversation to a close. 'Just one wig then. That will be £45.'

Outside it was still raining. I would have telephoned my husband for a lift but the hospital telephone box had been vandalized. In the end, I ran, with the push-chair, to take refuge in his office, four blocks away. When he asked how I had fared, and I started to tell him, I found to my dismay that I was tired and drab and practically in tears.

They had told me, these experts, that 'real human hair' wigs were the best, the most expensive, would appear most 'natural'. Respecting their expertise, I duly took my hospital prescription form to the wigmaker named.

The director of the firm was young, although the description of his company – makers of high-class wigs and postiche – had a quaint and elderly ring to it. This man was thirtyish, slim-suited, trousers taut over muscular thighs. He was gentle. Would I mind removing my scarf? He spoke softly, as though he knew it was like asking me to strip.

I fumbled clumsily with the scarf, so that he could measure the ugly, bare scalp. As my headscarf slipped to the floor, his expression changed. When he looked at me now, the mild approval I usually saw in male eyes had gone. This man had only one thing on his mind now: pity. Poor chap. With no hair and a huge expanse of moth-eaten scalp, I obviously looked like something from outer space. I wanted to show him a photograph taken a few weeks before. 'Hey, look, this is the real me!' I felt apologetic, uncharacteristically humble. I was reminded of the Nazis, shaving the heads of their Jewish women prisoners, of people's courts in France after the war, scalping the Germans' French mistresses. Always for the same reason: to humiliate.

**FACT: Bald People no Longer Feel Attractive. Their
Self-Image Too Often Goes Down the Drain With
Their Hair.**

My real hair wig cost me and the National Health Service
between us over £200. It took two months to make, needed
as much hairdressing attention as natural hair and had to be
sent away to be chemically cleaned. If I had been skilful with
it, it would no doubt have been ideal but when I arranged it,
I bore a close resemblance to a Buckingham Palace guards-
man. It ended up discarded at the back of the wardrobe.

My hairdresser bought me a pretty headscarf for my
birthday. That's when you've really hit trouble, I thought,
when your hairdresser buys you a scarf! Being a friend as
well as a hairdresser, she marched me off to the nearest
department store, where acrylic wigs were displayed in the
middle of the ground floor. Surrounded by shoppers, I was
aware of being noticed. Several knew me as a regional television presenter; a few nudged each other to point out 'what's-
her-name on the telly'. Usually I didn't mind, enjoying my
small local fame, but today I definitely did not want to be
recognized.

A pretty young assistant, with tactlessly flowing locks of
her own, yanked my scarf off in full view of — it seemed to
me — most of the world. She crammed on my head a thick
mass of 'mod acrylic' curls.

'Beautiful', declared my hairdresser. 'Washable at home,'
said the assistant. Lightweight, fashionable, practical for holidays . . . I hardly looked at myself in the mirror. I felt like
Danny La Rue in drag, as if the entire population was in the
store, laughing at me. 'You can even wash it in washing-up
liquid,' the salesgirl was enthusing. I wasn't listening, just
thinking of myself as 'that funny old woman who wears a
wig!' I wanted to escape, quickly.

I paid for it, without looking at any other styles, and rushed out. My friend had tried to persuade me to 'go home in it', so I squashed it under a scarf and hoped to get home before I met anyone I knew.

Once home, I pushed the acrylic wig, with the first one, into the back of the wardrobe. A disgraceful waste of money. Hysterical behaviour. Too right.

FACT: To a Bald Woman a Wig is a Prosthesis not a Fashion Accessory.

Wig manufacturers have for too long ignored the embarrassment of bald female customers trying on wigs in the middle of the ground floor of a crowded store. Now at last they are improving their service and offering a curtained-off dressing cubicle. They are also offering postal sales. But I didn't know that then.

Back into scarves I went, more or less round the clock. But you can't wear a headscarf forever. After about six months I returned to the store and was lucky enough to find another – more sympathetic – salesgirl. No hard sell this time. Quietly spoken and tactful, she found me a corner in the staff cloakroom where I could try on wigs in peace.

This one looked good, better than my own hair had ever done. I was so pleased with it. I left the store wearing it, admiring my reflection in shop windows.

With such newly found 'glamour' I was even confident enough to go back to the studios. But no light is brighter, no lens more ruthlessly truthful than in television. The TV camera never lies, except to add a couple of stones in weight to anyone foolish enough to stand in front of it. It would have been much easier to get away with a wig if I had been appearing on the stage. In the live theatre, Leichner make-up lines are harder and colours more garish. The stage is a long way from the audience. Television close-ups are really close. You can't disguise one single hair slipping out of place. So what chance did I have of fooling the viewers? I had no choice, however. Who can afford to sit at home moping indefinitely in a headscarf?

So back I went and appeared weekly, bewigged, before 10 million viewers. I did not mention it on the programme. 'Let them think you've got a sudden penchant for wigs,' said my best friend. 'After all, half of the actors in *Dallas* and lots of people in the English soap operas are wearing wigs. Why not you?'

If the viewers spotted it, they weren't rude enough to say so, not directly anyway. A few people quizzed the programme secretary. There was usually a question they had been dying to ask and did she mind . . . they weren't being rude . . . but was my hair false? That was the pattern. People asked my workmates, they rarely put the question to me.

I soon realized that my colleagues also knew. Their silence confirmed it. No one ever mentioned hair any more. No one said, 'Your hair looks nice' or 'Your hair looks a mess!' At first I kidded myself that no one would notice but their silence said: 'We're not stupid.' They knew.

Outside the studios, I could easily tell when people suspected. In the middle of a conversation their 'eye line' – the line of direct eye-contact – would be raised to the top of my head, then they would quickly, guiltily, look back into my eyes. Just a flicker, but it revealed that they knew, though nothing was ever said.

At home, convinced that my husband would never find me attractive again, I took to wearing wigs permanently, even in bed. Pathetic, really, I suppose. I looked so revolting with my moth-eaten bald head that it was only kind to both of us to hide it as much as possible. But wigs are hot and sticky. Many a night I would be scuttling down the landing to take it off and fumble for a scarf. It didn't do the wigs much good either. They got tangled and matted, but I felt better.

Sent home by the dermatologist in the vague hope that my hair would grow back of its own accord, I could only attempt to be patient – but I was lonely and couldn't find a support group. So I wrote my magazine feature and listed the horrors of alopecia areata.

- You are suddenly a freak, more a monster from outer space than a normal person. You've lost not only your hair but your eyelashes and eyebrows as well.
- Many doctors seem embarrassed and helpless. They are much happier treating the patients they know how to help than those who are suffering from an ailment which many consider 'purely vanity'.
- No one knows whether you will be bald for life. In a third of cases the hair does grow back spontaneously, but you can only hope you are going to be one of the lucky ones.
- Baldness is funny, a joke to everyone but you.
- You feel inexplicably ashamed and spend your life hiding your head.
- You get the impression from everyone around you that it is in some way your own fault. You are 'hysterical'. You are 'imagining things'.
- You are an unnecessary burden on the hospitals, where staff ought to be treating those who are really sick.
- You are a bit odd, peculiar, different.
- You are on your own. It has never happened to anyone else. That's how I felt. But there, as it turned out, I was wrong.

2

WHAT CAUSES ALOPECIA?

'I was not alone . . . far from it!'

I had received many letters after my magazine feature appeared but I was unprepared for the avalanche of mail which came in after my programme for BBC Radio Four's *Woman's Hour*. All the letters came from people desperate for help. They wrote of lives disrupted by baldness. Wives described hiding their patchy or completely bald scalps, even from their husbands. A pretty 'blonde' from the Home Counties told me, 'I hide my wigs from both my husband and my daughter. It is an effort but I'm sure they don't know.' Male sufferers were equally unhappy.

ROBERT, a bank executive whose alopecia started when he was a child in Canada, said: 'I know I look ridiculous. People laugh when they see me. They try to smother their amusement and giggle behind their hands. Some think I'm wearing a wig because I'm a punk rocker.

'A middle aged woman was whispering in the street the other day. She and her daughter were behind me on a crossing. I usually put up with this sort of thing and don't say anything, but this time I turned around and said to the mother: "Perhaps you'll lose your hair one day!"'

***CLARE**'s letter was an urgent appeal for help. 'I am in my thirties and have suddenly lost most of my hair. I feel at a complete loss. My life has had to change. My social life has gone, along with my confidence and some friends. My husband and I feel it is putting a strain on our marriage and I feel it's all my children's fault as it only happened after they were born. Why has this happened to me?'*

There was that sixty-four thousand dollar question again. When it first happens, this is the question we all ask.

Clare was obviously so upset that I found myself in the car on the way to see her straight away.

She lived in a pretty new house in a Cotswold village. It was the kind of family which might win a prize for twentieth-century contentment: husband in a good professional post in the nearest town, two children. Clare was a young woman of spirit, given to organizing community events, caring for the village elderly and raising money for playgroups. Her house had always had a welcome for other people's children as well as her own – until now. Suddenly Clare had stopped being sociable. She no longer invited people to the house, often failed even to answer the front door bell. Sometimes she screamed at the children. That day she had smacked her daughter, aged 3, too hard. The child was crying; so was Clare.

'I feel that any minute I'm going to snap. I'm terrified I'm going to become a baby-batterer. My husband comes home and sees me going bananas and thinks I've really gone mad.'

Eight weeks after the birth of her second child, a son, her life had been torn apart. In the bath with her 3-year-old daughter, she had been hurt when the child said, 'I don't want to have a bath with you any more, Mummy. There's too much hair in the water.'

It was true. Hair was falling out everywhere. Within a few

weeks the bald patches had spread, almost taking over Clare's scalp. She felt strange. Something peculiar had happened to her. She explained: 'When a man loses his hair he can walk down the street and feel macho. When a woman loses her hair — you look in the mirror and think "My God, what on earth can I do?" You just don't feel normal.'

Why Did It Happen To You?

Worrying about why it should have happened is one of the worst things in those early days. As it is very unlikely that anyone can give a satisfactory reason, I always advise against wasting too much time brooding about possible causes. Alopecia baffles even the experts, so it is pretty pointless to try to work out why. It's rather like asking 'Why did I catch flu?'

But some evidence is available. These are the clues I received when I asked that important question, 'why?'

Is It a Symptom of Something More Serious?
Hair loss may possibly be caused by a major medical disorder. The first thing a doctor will check is whether this is likely in your case. Blood tests should establish whether you are low on iron, possibly anaemic.

Hair loss may also be caused by a disorder of the thyroid, the endocrine gland which controls the body's metabolism through its secretion thyroxine, or it could be related to other conditions, such as diabetes, heart disease or disorders of the liver.

The chances are that all these conditions will be quickly eliminated. Then you will be back with the mystery. You are lucky enough to be perfectly healthy in every other way. You have 'only' lost your hair. Why?

Is It Because I'm a Neurotic?

Am I the type of personality the doctors label 'hysterical'? We all know the 'neurotic personality' – or think we do! He or she may appear quite calm, but underneath there is a mass of conflict and repression. This is a person who is under stress and it has been suggested for many years that stress causes the hair loss.

Over and over again, alopecia victims have told me: 'I'm sure the doctor thinks I'm neurotic.' Sarah, a hospital sister who lost all her hair, said, 'My GP just dismissed me as "hysterical".'

For years it was the standard answer in alopecia. Stress was such an easy explanation. Around the world, patients sat humbly in doctors' surgeries and got the distinct impression that he thought it was all in the mind. When it first happened to me, I realized very quickly that, though the medics were not actually saying so, they had a strong feeling that I was 'unstable'. Surely I must be or my hair wouldn't have fallen out! They were too kind, too polite to voice it, but I could tell. There I was, in their eyes, not only bald but bonkers! No wonder I didn't want anyone to know.

Doctors used to be sure of the link between alopecia and stress. It was well documented in the archives of medical research. Or was it? It is only recently that the medical profession has begun to question the link. If you look closely at the 'evidence' for stress you find that it is very flimsy indeed.

Until the 1950s, there were many reports from individual doctors of alopecia apparently triggered by stress but when psychiatrists tried to test this theory by using standard psychiatric procedures, they found it very difficult to prove. The 'evidence' depended on inconclusive research into a tiny number of cases and was directly contradicted and dismissed by an authoritative British psychiatrist more than 30 years ago.

It boils down to this: *You may have alopecia but you are probably no more hysterical than anybody else.*

By the time you have done the rounds of the GPS and dermatologists you will know by that look in their eyes that they are wondering about your psychological state. Just what flaw in your make-up has made you incapable of coping with life's normal care-load?

Your doctor may ask:

- Has there been any stress in your life recently?
- Have you recently had a life crisis, a family bereavement, moved house or lost your job?
- Is your marriage happy?
- Are you a worrier, prone to fretting about the smallest of problems (the kind of worrying that psychiatrists label 'free-floating anxiety', where your fears attach themselves to the nearest thing, no matter how trivial)?
- Are you an achiever, desperate for success and recognition, programmed from birth by ambitious parents?

If you answer yes to any of these questions, you may be suffering from stress.

Stress is thought to affect the hair follicles. These pouches contain the root of the hair and the papillae, the vital capillaries linking the body's blood supply to each growing strand of hair. It is thought that stress affects the hair follicles by constricting the blood vessels which feed them and so limiting their supply of oxygen.

Consultant dermatologist Dr Rodney Dawber of the John Radcliffe Hospital, Oxford, co-author of the definitive textbook on scalp disease, is one of the most distinguished men in the field.³ He explains: 'Stress is an important factor in some cases but in many it appears to play no part at all.' Alopecia areata has, for many years, been considered a trophoneurotic condition, a 'nervous' disorder only in that the patient's system was failing to provide adequate nutrition to the hair follicles, a condition governed by nerves.

'Over the years,' says Dr Dawber, 'attempts have been made to evaluate the role of stress in alopecia by using standard psychiatric procedures. The results have been, to say the least, contradictory.' In 1955, an Italian research team used standard psychiatric procedures to show that over 90 per cent of patients with alopecia areata were psychologically abnormal.⁴ Three years later a British psychiatrist, Dr I. Macalpine studied 125 patients with this disorder and came to the conclusion that emotional factors did not play a significant part.⁵

'Most of us working in the field would go along with Dr Macalpine's report,' says Dr Dawber, 'but there are still cases where emotional stress appears to have triggered the first attack.'

Psychologists have suggested that people with alopecia are the type who suffer feelings of inferiority and need encouragement. The chances are that if they aren't feeling inferior and low-spirited before their hair falls out, they certainly feel like this afterwards as a direct result of this depressing and disfiguring disease.

If alopecia is an auto-immune disorder it is still possible that it could be triggered by a period of stress. An episode of alopecia would normally occur up to four months afterwards. A complication is that if you suggest to someone that they have been under stress, it is pretty well certain they'll come up with some example. But many people declare that they were perfectly happy at the time it happened.

BARRY, *29, who describes himself as 'the eternal optimist, take-life-as-it-comes kind of chap,' underwent a period of stress when he lost his job in industry at a time when he had a new wife, a new mortgage and a new baby on the way. He had heavy financial worries. Finally his marriage broke up in what he describes as a 'messy' divorce. Through that period, his hair grew normally.*

Now the trauma is over. He has a job and his life is stable again, but he is rapidly losing his hair in the characteristic patches of alopecia areata.

'I can't understand it,' he says. 'It would have made more sense if I'd lost my hair during all that domestic hassle. The only other time I can remember losing any hair was when I was a teenager taking A levels. The patch was so tiny I hardly noticed it and it cleared up easily.'

NICK, *28, an RAF sergeant serving in Germany, started to lose his hair at a time when he was very pleased with himself. He had just won a car in a competition.*

Other cases link up directly with stress or shock.

JOHN, *35, a printer, started to lose his hair when his wife was in hospital dying of breast cancer. 'It was 18 months between the diagnosis of cancer and her death. She was only 40 and I was left with two children. My hair came out in patches from the moment the doctor told me the terrible prognosis. Losing my hair was nothing, of course, compared with the tragedy of my wife's death. Now my hair loss is total and I have to wear a wig.'*

ANITA *was 13 when she came home to discover her father in the bath in the middle of a suicide attempt. 'He had cut his wrists and ankles and stabbed himself,' she says. 'I bandaged him up, called an ambulance and went with him to hospital. A few months later I started to lose my hair. I had two years of misery until I left school and was able to wear a wig "full time" instead of just at weekends.'*

The alopecia seemed to clear up but eight years ago she had some patches after each of her two children's births. The hair grew back quickly.

Anita is now 33. 'Up to two weeks ago I was a contented married woman with a super husband and two lovely children aged eight and six. I didn't think I was under stress nor have I had any major shocks. So I was totally devastated when I saw a bald patch on the top of my head. Several others followed a few days later.'

So Anita has now suffered from alopecia areata over a period of 20 years. Sometimes the episodes seemed to be triggered directly by stress, at other times not at all.

Says Dr John Wilkinson, consultant dermatologist at the Wycombe General Hospital, High Wycombe: 'The progress of this condition is so eccentric that it is better not to say "My hair is back and it is over" but always to say that it is on an "up" phase (i.e. growing in) or a "down" phase. You can never relax!'

The debate as to whether it is caused by stress has been going on for years, almost since alopecia areata was first reported, back in Roman times. Since then, it has also been linked with everything from bad stomachs to bad teeth!

One of the oldest 'stress' case histories is that of the convicted murderer who was retried and reprieved several times by American courts. When he was under sentence of death his hair fell out; when he was reprieved it grew back . . . each time!

Is It Related to My Asthma or Eczema?
If you suffer from asthma or eczema as a family trait this puts you in the medical category labelled 'atopic'.

Many cases of alopecia areata occur in people who are atopic. Research figures have found this to be true in as many

as 50 per cent of cases.[6] This seems to vary in different parts
of the world. In a North American study, eczema or asthma
or both were present in 18 per cent of children with alopecia
areata and in 9 per cent of adults.[7] But in Japan, only 10 per
cent of patients were atopic.[8]

You are not more likely to suffer from alopecia areata if
you are atopic, but if you do suffer from this combination,
the prognosis is not good, particularly in a child.

When so much painstaking medical research has been
done, it may seem astounding to most of us that the doctors
are still baffled by the cause. Many patients are offered no
treatment, in their own interests.

Dr Dawber sees this as sometimes the best way to cope
with it. 'If the prognosis is poor – for example, if a child under
the age of puberty has a total loss of hair and is atopic – then
help in adjusting to the problems of wearing a wig will be of
far greater value to the child than the raising of false hopes.'

Did I Lose My Hair Because I Had a Baby?
Many women report that they went bald following a pregnancy.

Dr Joe Jordan, consultant obstetrician/gynaecologist at
the Queen Elizabeth Hospital, Birmingham, has seen quite
severe cases of hair loss among his patients. 'I am convinced
that it is due to a hormone swing,' he says.

It is, of course, well known that hair loss after a pregnancy
happens in 45 per cent of cases. Usually this clears up within
six months and the hair returns to normal, but many women
who contacted me had found that their problem was much
more serious. They had lost their hair severely – some totally
– soon after childbirth.

Medical opinion maintains that it is a question of defining
the different types of alopecia. Dermatologist Dr David

Fenton, who runs the Hair and Nail Research Unit at St Thomas's Hospital, London, which specializes in alopecia cases, told me, 'Alopecia areata does not normally start after a pregnancy. It is probably another type of hair loss such as telogen effluvium, diffuse thinning or even androgenetic (male pattern) baldness.'

As I have already reported, my own 90 per cent hair loss was considered by my GP to be linked with a pregnancy 15 months earlier, but the consultant dermatologist who saw me flatly rejected this theory and diagnosed 'classic alopecia areata'. A second consultant dermatologist labelled it 'diffuse alopecia areata'.

Dr Michael Sheppard, professor of endocrinology at Birmingham University, says, 'A new possibility is that a high proportion of women suffer an episode of thyroid dysfunction in the six to twelve months after giving birth. This could cause their hair loss but be missed in diagnosis, because of the time lapse involved in a referral from a GP to a hospital consultant. By the time a woman has a blood test for it, the thyroid will be back to normal. But the damage, in terms of hair loss, has already been done.

'Studies in Japan, North America and the UK have found that 10 per cent of women in the UK get a thyroid dysfunction after childbirth – about 5 to 6 per cent in the other countries. This could well trigger hair loss.

'This may be the reason a woman loses her hair after childbirth but she may never know.'

Often, alopecia patients report that their hair grows back in pregnancy, but falls out after the birth.

While many women, including myself, will report that they had no episodes of alopecia *at all* until after pregnancy, there are many who have suffered tiny bald patches earlier in their lives, perhaps no bigger than a 10 pence piece. Sometimes a small patch goes unnoticed. Then, once a baby is born, the mothers have a lot more bald patches, even to the extent of losing all scalp and all body hair. This is what happened in Clare's case.

CLARE *had had a small episode of alopecia when she was 14, at a time when her parents were divorced. Another tiny patch came at 20 when her mother was very ill, but these soon cleared up.*

She had no further problems, even when she had her first child, a girl. Then, because alopecia areata is an eccentric disease, she started losing hair heavily after the birth of her second child.

'I didn't worry when my little girl first pointed it out because I thought it would clear up as quickly as the first time,' said Clare, 'but soon my hairdresser pointed out the patches. My doctor said "It's alopecia. Nothing to worry about. Go home. Forget it." But you can't. It's such a frightening thing.'

Her husband joked: 'I would still love you even if you had no hair at all!' Soon, it was apparent that this was no joke. For a while they could hide it. When they visited their parents, her husband would walk down the drive behind her, to make sure her scalp wasn't showing through the thinning hair.

Every night television commercials glorified hair. Models had long, flowing, blond waves; Clare had not even enough to cover her scalp. She donned a scarf and hid in the kitchen. As her sitting room has large picture windows overlooking the road, passers-by can easily look in, so Clare began to stay in the kitchen most of the time.

She was lonely: 'I can't bear to meet people. This is not an illness you can talk about, like bronchitis or having your appendix out. I worry most about "taking it out" on the children. We both wanted them so much, especially as at one time we had an infertility problem and thought we might never have any. But when this happened, I blamed them. I thought that I would not have lost my hair if I hadn't had children'.

In fact, Clare's alopecia had really started many years before with that tiny patch at 17. When she underwent the trauma of childbirth it certainly seemed to cause her alopecia to flare up again – but only with the second pregnancy, not the first.

Will Another Pregnancy Make My Alopecia Worse?

The progress of alopecia areata is so erratic that this question is impossible to answer. As in Clare's case, you may lose hair after one child, but not another. This makes a nonsense of planning a family around it. Most women regard having children as the priority, having hair as a lesser – if desirable – consideration.

JANET, a service wife in the Middle East, lost a small patch of hair at 17. It followed the death of her father and her own involvement in a road accident. She seemed to lose more hair, in patches, when she was in her twenties and taking the oral contraceptive pill.

Stationed with her husband in Germany, she stopped taking the pill and for a while her hair improved. She had her first child and breast-fed for six months. As soon as she stopped breast-feeding, the hair fell out again, this time severely, and she had to resort to a wig.

SUE, aged 36, who lives near Dungeness power station where her husband works, had experienced one patch at the age of 8. This seemed to be related to emotional problems at school over a teacher she disliked. Then she had no hair problems until she started a family. In her first labour, the child's umbilical cord threatened his life. The second birth was also difficult and was followed by a serious haemorrhage. Soon after that, large bald patches spread into each other, leaving only a 'Friar Tuck' fringe, then it became total hair loss.

Over and over again, women contact me to report that their hair loss seemed to start with a pregnancy, without any previous occurrence. These are severe cases of more than 70 per cent hair loss, not merely the normal hair loss associated with pregnancy.

CAROL, *wife of a policeman, lost most of her hair when she was 23. Her baby was 11 months old and, like Janet, she had just stopped breast-feeding. 'I could only imagine that the changes in my body which the end of feeding meant, had triggered my hair loss. I wasn't under any stress and had a very understanding and loving husband.'*

ELIZABETH's *heavy mane of silky dark hair was her pride and joy, but it started to come out in big patches when her second child was a year old.*

A cheerful, attractive country woman who idolized her children, Elizabeth suggested to her doctor that her pregnancy had been responsible and was assured, 'No. This is a different type of alopecia. That it happened after a pregnancy is purely coincidental.'

'There was definitely no sign of baldness before the babies,' said Elizabeth. 'The only thing I could think of which might have caused it was a long period of worry the previous year when my mother was dying of cancer. Then my father-in-law had a stroke and we were obviously concerned about him. But of course we can all find stress in our lives if we think about it!'

Another important factor in the cases of both Carol and Elizabeth is that they are atopic. Both have asthma and eczema, which runs in their families. Carol suffered from it mainly in childhood but Elizabeth gets eczema and bouts of asthma quite severely. She suffered prolonged attacks a week or so after giving birth, on both occasions.

HILARY's *hair loss started out of the blue after childbirth. She does not remember an earlier episode of alopecia but knows that her* *mother had severe asthma. She wrote to me: 'I have been wearing a headscarf for 13 years.'*

A drab woman, I imagined, dowdy and old before her years. I was wrong. The tall, slim woman who met me at the station was sun-tanned and beautiful. Her headscarf was a blue silk Liberty print, swathed elegantly around her smooth shoulders.

Married to an industrialist, Hilary found that her hair had started to fall out after her first child, a daughter. 'At first I thought it was merely normal hair loss after giving birth until it became apparent that it was somewhat greater than normal.

'I sought advice everywhere and attended a local hair specialist — a trichologist — after the doctors just didn't seem to know! Then the hair began to grow again and I felt terrific.'

But Hilary wanted another child. 'I didn't want Rachel to be an only one and the trichologist did warn it might happen again. After Kate's birth, of course, it did.'

This time Hilary lost a lot more hair. 'I was sent to the skin clinic of a London hospital but the gentleman I saw was of the opinion I looked healthy and certainly wouldn't die of my complaint. Little did he know! When this happens, your self-confidence dies within you. Without my husband, my smashing little girls and my friends' support, I would have fallen apart. He was right, I wasn't going to die. But I died inside.'

Is the Pill Responsible for My Hair Loss?

Yes, in many cases. When you ask your doctor he is likely to say, 'No. The pill is the most widely taken, well-researched drug in medical history. Don't you think we would have discovered it by now if it was causing hair loss?' Or he may say: 'Nonsense. The pill can only improve your hair.' True — with some types of contraceptive pill, but many types of pill actually trigger hair loss.

It may come as a shock to those of us who were 'brought

up' on the pill, who swallowed it cheerfully for years as the easy, convenient answer to all our birth-control problems, but the fact is simple: the pill can make your hair fall out. The culprit? Progestogen, the synthetic hormone contained in the pill. Two progestogens – norgestrel and norethisterone – account for the progestogen component of the vast majority of oral contraceptives.

Doctors in Britain, West Germany and California, USA, have discovered that some women on pills with these components develop acne vulgaris, hirsutism or scalp hair loss. They either come out in spots, grow too much hair where they don't want it or go bald! Researchers at University College and St Mary's Hospital, London, reported these 'detrimental effects' in some women in 1979.[9] This report followed the research of endocrinologists in West Germany five years earlier, which listed the same effects in some women.[10] The two progestogens which caused the acne vulgaris, hirsuties or scalp hair loss were norgestrel and norethisterone acetate, which are contained in the majority of contraceptive pills, combined with mestranol or ethinyl oestradiol. The progestogen-only pills contain them exclusively.

They had an androgenic effect – an effect of male hormones – on some women. They lowered the level of Sex Hormone Binding Globulin (SHBG). This is the serum or plasma protein dependent on the oestrogen/androgen balance. It is used as a suitable biological marker of these properties in a woman. The woman with a low level of SHBG is likely, for instance, to suffer severe pre-menstrual symptoms. The problems occurred when a woman who already had a low SHBG level, plus a family tendency towards male pattern baldness, was put on a pill containing these particular progestogens. She then ran a high risk of losing her hair.

But have we only just discovered that the pill can trigger hair loss?

No, it has been suspected for years. In 1968, Dr S. R. Stephens reported in the *Journal of the Arkansas Medical Society* that when hair loss occurred in women on the pill it resembled the hair loss of the balding male. An androgenic effect was suggested as the cause. In 1979, Professor Vera Price pointed out that women who are predisposed to androgenic alopecia – hereditary thinning similar to male pattern baldness in a male – are the ones who notice the onset of diffuse thinning while taking some contraceptive pills.[11] She blames those progestogens whose metabolites have androgenic effects i.e. they cause baldness in the male pattern.

Dr Katharina Dalton, a world authority on the premenstrual syndrome, has long waged war on the progestogen content of the pill. She says: 'When it was introduced no one wanted to admit to women that they were being given male hormones. Women don't know the risks they take with the pill. Neither do their doctors. Over the years, they have found it easier to listen to the pill manufacturers, who would probably buy them a nice lunch, than pay attention to the evidence against it.

'The mechanism which causes hair loss is simple. Target cells in certain parts of the body, including the brain and the hair follicles, need natural progesterone which they receive through the receptor cells. Hair follicles need progesterone to help them develop. But the progestogens are artificial and do not give them what they require, so hair loss is the result.'

The suspicion has been there for many years. In 1967 American Dr Frank E. Cormia noticed that some women on the pill developed male pattern alopecia, and some had hair loss when they stopped taking the pill. Among German women in 1972, researchers reported that contraceptive pills with a high content of progestogen sometimes induced male pattern baldness in women who were predisposed to it.[12] Shortly, afterwards, Dr W. A. D. Griffiths of St John's Hospital, London, conducted a clinical investigation into the pill/hair loss debate.[13] While noticing that diffuse thinning did occur while women were on the pill, he concluded: 'There is no evidence to suggest that this is *because* they were taking oral contraceptives.'

LOUISE is a highly attractive woman in her early forties. She has a daughter. In the 1960s when she was in her teens and during the early years of her marriage, she was on one of the first oral contraceptives, with its 'heavier' formula of oestrogen and progestogen. Initially she was prescribed the pill for menstrual irregularities. 'I stopped taking the pill to start a baby,' says Louise, 'but I wasn't ovulating and had to have a pituitary stimulant to help me conceive.'

Some months after the birth, a large bald patch appeared on the crown of her head. 'Hair was falling out from all over my scalp. My doctor diagnosed alopecia areata and a rather unsympathetic dermatologist suggested I washed it too often.' Patchy baldness has now been a problem for twelve years.

Recently, she went to see a new dermatologist. 'I have also seen an endocrinologist and a trichologist to try to find some explanation,' adds Louise. 'My own feeling was that it all began with the pill. The dermatologist feels that there are several factors involved. It seems I have a predisposition to male pattern baldness. I am one of the unfortunate women whose hair follicles respond in some way to the androgen levels in my blood — exactly the same physiology as in common male baldness. The second factor was having a baby, followed by normal hair loss after childbirth. The third factor was that I had recently stopped taking the pill. These multi-factors combined were blamed for my baldness. The new dermatologist disputes the original diagnosis and says that this type of alopecia is definitely not alopecia areata.

At present my hair loss is not so bad that I have to wear a wig, but if it gets worse I am to go back to the dermatologist who may give me a course of anti-androgens.

I took the pill so happily all those years ago. It was the great liberator of my generation. But we were all guinea pigs. How was I to know I would go bald?'

So how is a woman to know whether taking the pill is triggering her hair loss?

Professor Michael Sheppard of Birmingham University says: 'As an endocrinologist, I see many women who are losing their hair. If they are on the pill, they ask: "Shall I stop taking it?" My advice is a three-point plan:

- Change the *type* of pill. You may find a different formula pill suits you better.
- If you are still losing hair, stop taking the pill altogether and use another method of birth control.
- If, after a reasonable period, you are still losing hair, then obviously the pill is unrelated to your condition and it doesn't make any difference to your hair whether you take it or not.'

But is there a contraceptive pill which does not trigger hair loss?

For patients with hair loss, especially those with common or male pattern baldness, it is important to choose a pill which does not make it worse.

Consultant endocrinologist Dr Christopher H. Mortimer: 'Pills which contain "androgenic progestogens" such as norethisterone, ethynodiol diacetate, lynoestronel or norgestrel should be avoided. I suggest a combination of ethinyl oestradiol with medroxyprogesterone acetate. Or Marvelon, a pill from Organon, may be suitable in certain cases.

Dianette, a pill sometimes given to women suffering from androgenic hair loss, is another possibility but probably not for routine use.'

I Suffer from PMT. Will I Lose My Hair if I Take the Pill?

You run that risk. The miserable symptoms of pre-menstrual tension (PMT) – or pre-menstrual syndrome (PMS) – including lethargy, bad temper, weepiness and weight gain, are often marked biologically by a lowering of Sex Hormone Binding Globulin (SHBG). If this shows up in blood tests, it is often the signal that a woman needs treatment for PMT.

A lowering of SHBG has been noticed among some women on the pill, so if you take it, you could be lowering SHBG even more and you may be more likely to suffer hair loss.

Many women who have lost their hair have reported to Hairline that their PMS symptoms grew worse at the same time.

HAZEL, a college lecturer in computer science, was baffled by the sudden loss of all her hair. She linked it immediately with pre-menstrual syndrome.

'At the time I was losing my hair – during that terrible "fall-out" phase – my behaviour in the days before menstruation became violent and erratic, but I was told at the hospital that blood tests to establish my connection would be long and involved. They would

have needed to know my hormone levels before the hair loss to come up with any valid findings.'

She is bewildered. 'I dream that I have hair again. The question I need answered is why?'

Could the Progestogen I Take for PMS Cause Hair Loss?

Women who suffer from PMS are often prescribed a progestogen to combat their symptoms.

HELEN, 32, *is convinced that her hair loss is related to the progestogen she has been taking for seven years. She started to lose her hair two years ago.*

'I didn't lose it all but most of the crown, front and sides went, like a man. I was forced to wear a wig. I used to sit at home feeling I looked like Queen Elizabeth the First!'

MARY, 35, *also relates her hair loss to the progestogen she takes for PMS. 'After the birth of my baby I started to feel so terrible in the days before my periods that I was afraid I would hurt the baby. I have severe symptoms for nearly a fortnight every month.'*

She has two children now, aged six and three, and has had several miscarriages. Her hair, healthy during pregnancy, has now fallen out at the temples and around her face. Her doctor has diagnosed male pattern baldness due to an over-sensitivity to androgens.

'I feel and look so terrible now with all this hair gone that I'm afraid it is wrecking my family life.'

But Do these PMS Progestogens Trigger Hair Loss?

'Yes,' says Dr Katharina Dalton. 'The progestogens cause a lowering of blood progesterone which the hair follicles need.'

'No,' says Michael Sheppard, professor of endocrinology at Birmingham University. 'There is no epidemiological evidence for this. So much research has been done on them that any evidence would have been uncovered by now.'

One of the most commonly used progestogens for PMS is dydrogesterone, which has been the subject of research at Guys' and St Thomas's Hospitals for many years. Dr Michael Brush, senior lecturer in reproductive chemistry, says: 'We have found no evidence that this progestogen has any effect on hair growth. Dydrogesterone can reduce blood progesterone by a mean of 15 per cent but what really matters is the total progestational activity of the progesterone and the progestational agent (i.e. dydrogesterone). The drugs are being used on a pharmacological level, i.e. a much higher level, and not at a physiological level.'

In other words, the drug floods the system with a far greater amount than required. The body uses as much as it needs and the surplus is excreted.

Could Natural Progesterone Help in Cases of Hair Loss?

Dr Dalton feels that if women who had lost hair in this way were given natural progesterone in high doses their hair might return – even several years after the original loss. *Natural* progesterone was originally extracted from animals' ovaries and is now manufactured from the roots of yams, whereas progestogen is the synthetic version. Natural progesterone cannot be taken orally as the body cannot absorb it properly, so it is administered by injection or as suppositories or pessaries.

Dr Dalton describes a case where hair regrew after treatment with natural progesterone.

'A 29-year-old married woman had total loss of scalp hair, which had started at the age of 7 as patchy alopecia areata. By the time she was 17 she needed a wig. Her hair improved miraculously during her two pregnancies, at 20 and 25, but when she went on the pill she became depressed and had marked deterioration in the alopecia. Six hormonal investigations were normal but she had a low SHBG level which suggested she might respond well to progesterone therapy.

'Six months after she started this therapy the hair was beginning to grow again. A year later, she had fair hair in the patchy areas and especially good hair in the front hair line. Two years after she started the treatment she was able to discard her wig and had a good covering of hair throughout her scalp. After another year she had a full head of dark ash-blonde hair.'

Is Hair Loss Caused by the Menopause?

It is known that the falling levels of female hormones which occur after the menopause can trigger diffuse thinning in women. Women often ask 'Would Hormone Replacement Therapy help my hair?' HRT, of course, eases other symptoms in these difficult years – eases hot flushes and panic attacks and also helps to prevent the brittle bones of osteoporosis. Doctors tell us that most women also find their hair improves too – except for the unfortunate few who are genetically predisposed towards thinning hair. For these, the progestogen (synthetic progesterone) component of HRT can have an androgenic effect on the hair and cause it to thin. For this reason, some doctors prescribe natural progesterone (Cyclogest) as an alternative to a progestogen. This is administered as a suppository or pessary.

In some cases the menopause can also herald severe alopecia areata, usually in patients who have had earlier, less severe episodes.

*JOAN, for instance, had suffered a small patch of alopecia areata
as a teenager, but she lost all her hair shortly after the menopause.
She was sure in her own mind that the two events were linked but her
doctor assured her that the menopause could not have been responsible. She says: 'I was told by the medical profession that the condition was neither hormonal nor psychological, but as they have no
idea of the cause I do not know how they can be so dogmatic.'*

Some doctors, however, think the menopause *might* be
involved in some types of balding.

*DOROTHY's dermatologist went along with her theory that it
had all started with the menopause. Tiny patches of alopecia had
begun when she was 47. She was also under stress as her husband
had recently lost his job. Her specialist put it down to 'a hormone
imbalance caused by the menopause and aggravated by stress.'*

It has been known for years that a certain type of hair loss –
often a rather sparse 'thinning' to the hair – occurs as
women grow older.

Does it Mean I'm Going Bald Like a Man?
Am I Less of a Woman Because of My Hair Loss?

Don't be offended if your doctor mentions common/male
pattern baldness. Alopecia androgenetica is merely another
type of hair loss in which the hair follicles respond, in exactly
the same way as balding men, to the androgen levels in the
blood. Both men and women have androgens – the male
hormones – in their make-up and an imbalance or oversensi-
tivity to these androgens can cause hair loss.

There are some rare virilizing conditions in women which
cause male pattern baldness where a woman develops addi-
tional masculine characteristics. These are very serious and

need the urgent attention of a good gynaecologist or endocrinologist, in case a tumour is involved.

There are also much milder versions of this, in which the woman is still feminine in appearance, can have children and live as normally as any other woman. She is merely a sufferer from an over-sensitivity to androgens which can cause her to lose hair in a similar pattern to a man. Some experts have suggested that women who are predisposed to this type of hair loss are the ones whose hair goes thin when they are on the contraceptive pill. It has also been suggested that these days more career women are suffering from male pattern baldness due to their recently acquired 'equality' with men. They are gaining the advantage of taking on jobs previously held by men only to find that they are also gaining men's health problems – coronaries, strokes and common baldness! Treatment with anti-androgen drugs is reasonably successful in such cases.

SANDRA is 32, the adopted daughter of an Australian doctor. She is studying in London. Tall, full-breasted, she is, as she puts it, 'a large lady'. She is 5 feet 8 inches tall and weighs 14½ stones. She lost most of her hair when she was 11, not in bald patches, but as a general thinning.

Her condition has been diagnosed as common/male pattern baldness. 'This hurt at first, but I know I'm a real woman because I have been pregnant,' says Sandra. 'I know I'm overweight but I'm what people used to describe as "comely"'.

Her hair now covers her head completely but is very thin, like baby down. 'People can see straight through to my scalp,' she says. 'A Brisbane taxi driver once dropped me with the farewell "Jesus, lady, but your hair is thin." I just want to look normal, get married, have children. I want ordinary hair. I often catch people looking at me as if to say "She's a funny bunny!" I used to work with the mentally ill. Maybe I thought I got away with being a bit of an oddball with them.'

She wears very smart clothes, tailored skirts and beautiful hats. 'I love hats and have now discovered the cocktail hat where a bow or a rose and bit of net can be placed strategically on the bald front of my scalp.

'Once I went for a job interview wearing a wig. I got the job and had to carry on wearing a wig for two years. But before I left I took it off and showed everyone my scalp. "This is the real me!" I told them all.

'I have a boyfriend at the moment. I got him through an ad in a singles magazine, where he was advertising for a "big girl". Well, I qualify there – my breasts grew to a 36B very early on. I often wondered whether it was too early and upset my hormones.

'Anyway this chap lived two hundred miles away so we met half-way and went on a dirty weekend, in a youth hostel, of all places, in separate dormitories! He says he doesn't mind about my lack of hair but whenever anyone comes to the door he says "Put your wig on quickly!"'

Sandra is now seeing an endocrinologist who has explained that treatment may take two years.

It has been suggested that her baldness is hereditary, but this is difficult to establish as she is adopted.

'Sometimes I think I'll end up single for the rest of my life. It takes a deep breath and a smile before I can take the plunge and take my hat off when I meet a new man.

'Once I made the ultimate sacrifice of shaving all my hair off in the hope that it would come back thicker. It didn't.'

Says Professor Michael Sheppard: 'The hormonal differences between men and women are not so clear-cut as one might imagine. Only a very slight imbalance can make a difference. A woman might lose the hair on her head in the same pattern of receding temples as a man, while hair grows on her arms and legs.

'There are three groups who suffer from hair loss; the genetically predisposed, those who have common or male pattern baldness and by far the largest group where we just do not know the cause.'

Is the Cause Sometimes Something Rather Odd?

It is very rare indeed for people to find out exactly what caused their alopecia. Just occasionally, there are odd happenings where it can be linked with a definite substance. Some of the most unlikely reasons for hair loss have been suggested by the patients themselves.

ROSS, a handsome ex-army officer who now teaches, suddenly lost every hair on his body, at the same time as developing painful, blotchy purple rashes on his chest and shoulders. He was able to trace it back to a chemical spray he had been using in his own garden and which was also in regular use at his school. His doctor gained the co-operation of the firm who manufactured it and made investigations.

PAULINE, a housewife in Chesterfield, Derbyshire, who had lost a large percentage of her hair over a period of 20 years, was delighted when all her hair returned, due, she thinks, to taking zinc tablets. She had seen them recommended in a magazine about natural remedies and purchased them from a health-food shop. Within a few weeks, her hair began to return. 'It took ages, of course, to regrow — the best part of a year,' she says, 'but I know it was a daily dose of 75 mg of zinc which started it off.'

The problem with any regrowth in alopecia areata is that it often occurs by itself, so you can never be absolutely sure it was your remedy which regrew it! But zinc is well recognized as being involved in hair growth. Some animals who are deprived of zinc lose their hair!

Dr Alan Stewart and Dr Stephen Davies, authors of

Nutritional Medicine (Pan, 1987) blame zinc deficiency in some cases of human hair loss, but reckon that it can be restored and grow again thickly if zinc is taken.

It may well be worth considering a zinc supplement if you have hair loss – zinc sulphate, amino acid chelate – many types are available in your health-food shop.

Dr Davies suggests a *lower* dose than that chosen by Pauline: 'Thirty to fifty mg taken at night when the stomach is relatively empty, so other foods don't interfere with its absorption. If any nausea occurs split it into two doses taken during the day.' Oral zinc supplementation is relatively safe and non-toxic, he says, but warns against taking too much. 'Don't over-supplement with zinc unless it is being monitored by a doctor, as excessive zinc can cause a copper deficiency!'

Zinc is contained in many foods including shrimps, egg yolks, chicken, potatoes and pork chops.

One woman who took zinc to improve her hair found that her nails had never been so strong! Zinc is also believed to help in cases of rheumatoid arthritis.

NANCY, a grandmother from the North of England, reported that zinc tablets were not doing much for her hair – she lost it 30 years ago – but had certainly improved her dermatitis. 'My legs have never been better. I bless the day I heard about Hairline! And you never know – I might be Lady Godiva yet!'

Survival Plan

You are losing your hair rapidly. The worst part is *now* when so much is falling out. You waste a lot of time gazing into the mirror in horror. You are indecisive. You don't know which shampoo to use . . . whether to use lacquer, colour tint or permanent wave . . . Yards of hair collect on your comb. You worry over every strand. This can easily become an obsession. I've even found myself tracing the grain on my polished dressing table, thinking it was hair. I've examined the molecular structure of hairs which turned out to be from my mohair sweater! Hair seems to be everywhere, except on your head! You can't believe that it is all going like this. You feel like screaming. Hang on. A certain amount of hair loss is normal. Everyone loses up to 140 hairs a day, as part of the normal growth replacement cycle. You may be imagining it. If you are sure you are not, go to your doctor straight away to decide between you just what sort of hair loss you have.

If it is post-pregnancy hair fall it will probably be a general diffuse thinning all over the head or baldness in the male pattern, i.e. at the temples and on the crown. It would normally occur within a few months of childbirth or following an abortion, the causes being both hormonal and the physical trauma your body has experienced.

If it is alopecia areata it is likely to start with small round patches, sometimes surrounded by tiny stumps, called 'exclamation mark' hairs. These are withered hairs broken off near the scalp. Regrowth of each patch normally starts with vellous fine white hairs, a covering of down like a baby's, while hairs of normal colour come later. Often a patch will regrow, then another will start. This pattern of regrowth and bald patches may be lifelong.

Will It Clear Up?
A third of all patients get just one small episode – perhaps one patch – and completely recover with no re-occurrence.[14] Another third experience a relapse six months after the first episode and recovery takes much longer. If hair loss is total, 20 per cent of all cases never recover from the first episode.

If he or she feels your condition is severe, your family doctor may refer you to a consultant dermatologist. He or she may carry out blood tests to eliminate thyroid, anaemia or other systemic factors as the cause. In the United Kingdom, the dermatologist will be able to authorize a National Health Service (NHS) contribution towards the cost of wigs. The NHS pays roughly half the cost. You pay a contribution ranging from £40 for a man-made fibre wig (usually acrylic) to £151 for a full bespoke human hair wig. There is no charge if the patient is still at school.

The dermatologist may offer you a scalp cream, perhaps a topical steroid such as Betnovate, or minoxidil solution to rub daily into your scalp (see chapter 7).

You may be told 'There is nothing we can do. Go home. Forget it. It will probably grow back.'

Maybe it will, but it will take a long time. I did as I was told – i.e. nothing – on the advice of a dermatologist. 'If the worst comes to the worst,' I consoled myself, 'I'll look for alternative help.' Three years later, I surveyed my bald head in the mirror and observed that the worst had very definitely come to the worst. I certainly still looked bald, although some little, fine hairs were growing all over my head. At this stage I decided I needed more help or I would be in wigs forever.

I sought a new dermatologist and found an enthusiastic young clinical researcher with a real interest in alopecia. Such men are rare. He prescribed minoxidil, sometimes combined with tretinoin lotion (retoinic acid). The acid makes the minoxidol fairly itchy and uncomfortable but for me it was worth it as some regrowth began.

If It Gets Worse

If you feel that your GP has wrongly sent you home, dismissing your case as mild, it is always worth going back so that he or she can see how much it has deteriorated. No one likes to pester a busy doctor, but the average GP is taught at medical school that someone worried about hair loss needs reassurance. So he or she duly reassures. And sometimes, sadly, hardly seems to notice that the patient's head is nearly bald!

TRISHA, 30, reported: 'The doctor told me: "Don't worry. It will grow back." I went home and it got worse. My husband said: "You'll have to see him again."

'This time the doctor said "What do you think I can do about it?" I told him I wanted to see someone else. The doctor said "I don't know what you think a dermatologist is going to do for you." He referred me to a specialist but the appointment was six months ahead. I saw red and went back to the doctor. He gave me tranquillizers.'

The appointment was brought forward but by the time Trisha saw a specialist she had lost all her hair.

Even when you do see a dermatologist he or she may offer you no treatment if the prognosis is good. If the hair loss is patchy, not total, if you are not atopic and did not suffer it first in early childhood, then the dermatologist could feel quite justified in 'leaving it alone to grow back by itself.' With a bit of luck . . .

At first, I went quietly home to wait for my hair to regrow. I met a friend I hadn't seen for a while. 'What have you been doing?' she asked chattily. The only reply I could offer was 'Waiting for my hair to grow.' A bit negative, to say the least!

If You Have Tried to Obtain Conventional Medical Help and Failed. . .

. . . then you can look elsewhere, but be *careful* where you look. *Don't* spend a fortune on unlikely commercial clinics. The high street is full of them, so are the newspapers. Use your common sense. If they want £1,000 now, they'll want another £1,000 in three months' time when they've 'prepared the scalp' and got it 'ready for the treatment'. Have nothing to do with them. Heed these awful warnings:

MICHAEL, a young graphics artist, answered a newspaper ad. He booked an appointment at a so-called 'clinic' in a city over 100 miles away. He and his mother travelled from the West Country only to find that a 'consultant' — he was not a doctor — offered Michael a six-month course of treatment at a cost of £1,000. They gave him a trial treatment: a five-minute scalp massage and application of an unidentified lotion. A free hairbrush was thrown in. Their charge? £50.

'The sales pressure was so determined that we practically had to fight to get out,' says his mother. 'We ended up escaping with the promise of a further appointment. With our train fares, I reckon it cost us £100 — and the last thing Michael needed was a brush. He hasn't got much hair left to brush!'

EILEEN, 30, from Aberdeen, worried about her patchy alopecia areata, was tempted by a clinic's advertisement of an '80 per cent success rate' in regrowing hair. She went along for the promised free consultation.

'I was told I would have to visit them thrice-weekly for three to six months. The treatment would not start until I had paid them £1,250. They were very pushy and played on my misfortune. My doctor was appalled.'

With Eileen's husband unemployed and the family dependent on her job as a chemist, there was no question about her refusal.

ANDREW, *a TV salesman: 'As doctors couldn't help, I ended up in a clinic I saw advertised in a paper. They sold me a bottle of something which looked like vinegar and wanted £1,200 to start treatment. I refused it, but the clinic kept phoning and writing, badgering me to go back. They tried to sound sympathetic. One letter said "You must be feeling very distressed about your hair loss." I wrote back: "Not nearly as distressed as I would feel if I'd paid you £1,200." I heard no more.'*

All these stories show how easy it is to be tempted by the attractive promises of the commercial clinic and lose your money as well as your hair.

If you have given up on the medical profession, you could try a trichologist (hair specialist). But again, take care!

If you want a reputable trichologist, check with the Institute of Trichologists first (address, page 194). It operates from a modest 'hospital' in South London, but will give you the names of trichologists in your area.

Check how much the individual operator charges *before* you get there. If his or her premises are palatial, in the best part of town, the money to keep him or her there may well be coming from you. The average provincial trichologist's fee shouldn't break the bank. It should not be more than the price of a special hair-do, such as a blow wave, cut and conditioner.

One treatment a trichologist may offer you is electro-therapy – high-frequency electrical stimulation to the scalp. This works on the principle that blood circulation to the scalp is boosted, getting much-needed oxygen to the hair follicles. Some doctors say this is unnecessary but trichologists claim that it can make hair grow four times faster.

Mrs Jane Leddington, formerly lecturer in charge of the beauty department at Worcester Technical College, says:

'We teach our students to use high frequency and through it, I have seen cases of alopecia areata grow back. One man had gone bald over business pressures. With high frequency, his hair returned.'

MICHELLE, 16, from Gloucester, went to trichologist Mrs Barbara Kiddle for high frequency when her days at school were being ruined by patchy hair loss. Her hair gradually regrew.

Says Mrs Kiddle: 'Patients must allow six weeks before they see results. I've found it quite successful where women have thinning hair and possibly a tender scalp.'

But I Haven't Lost All My Hair.
How Do I Stop Any More Falling Out?
You can't. If alopecia areata is active, the condition is very difficult to arrest and better brains than ours are devoting years of research trying to do just that.

But you can make sure that what you put on it won't make it worse. Don't stand in the chemist's shop going cross-eyed over the countless hair products displayed. Usually the conditioners and shampoos sold by the big names in hairdressing will be best. You can buy those at the hairdresser's.

Many people point out that their hair would look thicker if they tinted it. This should do no harm if you choose a mild product. Be wary of permanent waves, however, as they generally mean applying a very strong chemical to the hair. You have to find a hairdresser you can trust and take advice on gentle products. Don't forget to condition the scalp as well as the skin on your face.

If Your Hair Is Thin
This may be due to losing a lot of hair in the patches of alopecia areata, or it may be gradual thinning which happens

after the menopause, or the 'male pattern' thinning of genetically predisposed people. Hair is there, for which you are thankful, but every time the sun shines or you stray under a spotlight you are aware that people can see straight through to your scalp.

Hairdressers' tricks can disguise it: back hair brought forward, no partings, especially centre ones, a bob style to cover thin patches, perhaps highlights on fair hair.

Modern mousses and thickening setting lotions also help. 'Hair loss is so common among women,' says Alexa Goodman, who runs salons in well-heeled Solihull, in the West Midlands, 'that we offer vitamin-based hair-thickening and hair-loss treatments. Some of these come from France, some from the big names in UK hairdressing.'

Wella make a hair thickening lotion – Cortex Corpus – which is applied on its own as a setting lotion and left on the hair while it is set or blow dried. A regular cut or trim is most important to prevent breakage. Having it cut will not stop it from growing as, if it has started to grow normally, it should grow at least half an inch every month.

Use only good quality combs and *bristle* hairbrushes. Plastic can stretch the hair and cause breakage and split ends. A gentle shampoo and regular washing with a good scalp massage will keep the scalp healthy, stimulate blood supply to the hair follicles and encourage growth.

Rules and Regulations
Don't raid the fridge or the drinks cupboard. Ban the words 'It's a shame to waste it.' I know you have a good excuse to overeat, feeling a bit sorry for yourself, and many alopecia victims do overeat to compensate. I did.

FACT: Getting Fat Makes It Worse.

The danger when you lose your hair is that you will not only eat too much but will also have a few drinks to go with it. An attractive night-club hostess, whose hair fell out after a hysterectomy, confessed: 'What could I do? I turned to the bottle.' Faces look fatter anyway in wigs. Take in extra drinks and the Bunter look is soon with us. If you eat too much and wash it down with one too many gins it won't be long before you end up not only bald but bloated – not the combination to bring lovers queuing ardently at your door!

You can't help being bald. You can help being fat, so don't be.

Do take up a sensible diet, high on fibre, low on fat, and get yourself some good vitamin supplements.

Make sure your diet is high in amino acids, the building blocks of protein which are found in meat, fish, eggs and dairy products. The amino acid L Tyrosine can be obtained in powder form through a pharmacy and trichologists recommend it for helping hair regain its normal colour. (See chapter 9 for more dietary tips.)

Don't listen to old wives' tales. There is always someone who knows exactly why it happened, who will blame you for all the tints and perms you had or some tablet you took. It's all claptrap. Ignore it.

Do shut up about it. To most people, the condition of someone else's hair is about as interesting as the dream they had last night. People don't understand anyway. They get embarrassed and behave as though you have had a death in the family. You have nothing to be ashamed of. You have just lost your hair. It is a scalp disease, not a social disgrace.

Don't worry. Now there's a daft suggestion. Who doesn't worry when their hair falls out in handfuls? But worrying really can prolong the problem. Try to relax, even if you have to go to relaxation classes to do it!

Don't panic.

Don't gaze at your hair frequently, obsessively, in mirrors.

Don't count hairs, as they come out, spread them out on white paper, or angle the looking glass so that you can glare at the back.

Do spend as much as you can afford on the beauty aids which will make you look and feel good, in spite of having no hair or only a little hair.

There are 101 ways to waste time worrying over alopecia. I should know, I've tried them all. You will not indulge in any of them. You will be too busy. You have positive things to do.

Not only will you survive alopecia, you will be successful, attractive and happy. You will look better than you've ever looked before. I promise.

PART II

VICTIMS

3

WHEN IT HAPPENS TO A WOMAN

*'Only if I know for certain that my husband is away
for the night will I sleep bareheaded.'*

Pauline, bald for 16 years, is married with a family of boys and
has a full-time teaching job.

*'I was left with a red scalp, bare and ugly, so I will not be seen
without a wig.'*

Roxanne is 36. Her hair finally departed totally after the birth of
her third baby, though she had had patchy hair loss since childhood.

*'I need a few drinks before I can sleep with my husband. Otherwise
I'm thinking, how can he want me when I look like this?'*

Kathleen has been bald for 45 years but still managed to land
herself two doting husbands. She has outlived them both.

*'You can't wear a wig in bed. Well, you can but the darned thing
keeps slipping off.'*

Hazel, 35, a small, elfin college lecturer, has been hairless for only
a year. She has been told by her doctor: *'You are likely to be bald for
life.'*

'Our families — the older generation — say "Poor Roger! He's got a

bald wife." They hate it when I won't wear a wig. But why should I? It's only to please other people. It's not like having to wear false teeth for the functional purpose of eating!'

Samantha, *36, has had alopecia since she was 3. Twice she has lost all her hair and then it has regrown. Now she has bald patches again.*

'Alopecia has affected me totally. My marriage has broken up. My husband is now living with someone else. It made me reclusive and unsociable. I couldn't bear him to see me. I used to go to bed in a scarf. I feel generally a total freak, ugly and unlovable.'

Stephanie *was 26 when her long auburn hair started to fall out. The attack was severe. 'I screamed and sobbed. I felt so ugly. I wouldn't let my husband anywhere near me sexually, so I suppose it wasn't surprising that he turned elsewhere. When I found out that he was cheating on me, I felt I just couldn't compete with another woman. So in the end he left me and we got a divorce. I can see now that I can't really blame my hair loss. It was the effect it had on me and the way I was behaving which really smashed us up.'*

'When I lost my hair it wrecked both my marriage and my career. I ended up alone in a strange city, broke, with nothing in the cupboard to eat.'

As Stephanie admits, it is how a wife copes with losing her hair which can make or break a marriage. In her case, her marriage was at risk before it happened.

The situation can be equally traumatic for a husband. In our society hair is a symbol of beauty and desirability. It is no coincidence that television commercials feature women with long wavy locks. So do fairy tales. Imagine Cinderella going bald!

For a successful intimate relationship, a woman needs self-esteem, to be in love with herself to some extent. It is not easy to make love when her mental self-image depicts a scalp which is patchy, moth-eaten or even completely bald.

CAROL, *23, a policeman's wife, says: 'Our sex life was badly affected. My hair took a year to fall out completely which was the worst time. Lots of hair coming out and just not knowing whether it was all going.*

'I felt such a mess I didn't think my husband could possibly want me sexually. In fact, sex came to a stop, possibly because I felt such a wreck and didn't want to — not because he didn't want me. He protested that he did. The hair loss made no difference. Once all my hair had gone I could just say "Well, it's happened and that's that." I've got used to the wigs now. I keep them on all the time, even in bed, because he doesn't like to see me without hair.'

LOUISE *was so shaken when she first lost some hair that she took a lover. She is attractive and knows it.*

'I'd always been vain, I suppose, sure of myself with men. After I lost some hair, I felt I looked frankly distasteful. My husband said it didn't matter. He hardly seemed to notice.

'I started an affair. It sounds as if I'm making my hair loss the excuse, but I had to find out whether men would still fancy me. This one did. He even reckoned he found my loss of pubic hair erotic!

'Of course it was disastrous. It got completely out of hand when he turned serious and wanted me to break up my marriage. Fortunately, I had the sense to get out of it without damaging my marriage and family.'

ANNA, *24, vivacious, long-legged district nurse, couldn't face the thought of marriage without hair. When she developed severe alopecia areata she cancelled her wedding. A slipped wig can put paid to many a moment of passion and Anna was afraid it would* happen to her. *'I wanted to be beautiful for my wedding. I couldn't face the thought of getting married without hair or in a wig. Not on this one special day.'*

Anna used to have long, wavy brown hair but she lost nearly all of it. She also lost her eyebrows and eyelashes.

She was engaged to an ambitious young accountant but her wedding preparations became fraught with problems. Her happy personality, which always charms the patients, somehow failed her when dealing with her fiancé's family. *'Everything I did was wrong. His mother insisted on taking over all the arrangements. She was very critical of me – my cooking, my clothes – and my fiancé didn't seem to defend me as I had expected. The bullying was getting me down, although I never show it when I'm worried. Deep down I was afraid it was all my fault.'*

She was also unhappy at work. She had been moved temporarily into a surgery job which did not involve seeing patients in their home, the part of the work she liked best.

A few months before the wedding date she started to lose her hair. Hair was blocking up the shower and seemed to be falling out steadily. A car accident was the last straw. *'I opened my eyes and I was lying on the pavement with people crowding around. In all the pain, blood and mess, all I could think about was my hair and whether these strangers could see how bald I was getting.'*

When she woke in hospital, nearly all her hair had gone. Anna made the decision to cancel the wedding. Her fiancé accepted it without question. *'He told me that my hair loss didn't make any difference. I was still Anna as far as he was concerned. But I think he felt guilty about my baldness. The doctor had blamed the family stress which I was going through, though personally I wondered whether it was connected with the pill.'*

For a while Anna and her fiancé continued to meet occasionally, *'But he kept letting me down. I was disappointed all the time.'* Now they never meet. Anna has tried to make new relationships but finds it a problem. 'I feel that all the men are looking at me and thinking that I'm wearing a wig.'

She no longer enjoys the preparation for a date. 'Getting ready used to be part of the fun of it. I haven't got eyelashes so I can't go putting on mascara and I haven't any eyebrows to pencil. Well, I could try but I feel too much like 'false part Annie' with false eyelashes, false eyebrows and the wig! Besides, I hate spending time looking in a mirror to make my face up. It's no longer a pleasure to me.'

She has carried on with her job and bought a wig for work. 'I have to look "normal" for the patients. There would be too many questions if I went to see them "bald". As it is, they often compliment me on my "pretty hair".'

Once at home, though, it's off with the wig and into a baseball cap for the rest of the day. In denims, with cap perched precariously on her ears, Anna looks like a cheerful pixie.

Her good humour is strictly for company. 'When I'm alone in the flat at night, I often start to feel really awful. I think my life is suspended until I get my hair back and goodness knows when that will be, if at all!'

The thought of a life without her hair is something which hits Anna when she is at her lowest. She thinks of killing herself as the solution. 'When I'm feeling down and low I contemplate suicide and it's like a safety valve. I think I'll give it another year or so then if my hair hasn't grown back I'll put an end to the misery of it all, because it's like a great heavy weight on you which stops you leading a normal life like any other young woman. I know it's weak. There are people much worse off than me, crippled, or in pain. I see it every day. But when you are down you don't think as logically as that.'

KATHLEEN has been living with baldness for 45 years, unlike Anna, for whom the problem has only just begun. She began to lose *her hair at the age of 6. She lived in a Welsh mining village, where she says, 'the minds were as narrow as the valleys'. One neighbour, from the chapel, told her mother it was unfair on the other children for her to go to school.*

'The worst thing for me was the isolation. Whereas my contemporaries could socialize, who would want to be seen with me — with or without a hat? When I was at teacher training college I couldn't really enjoy the wartime dances like everyone else. I used to dance with the RAF men who were stationed near the college, but I stayed remote.

'My sex life had to be restricted as I never wanted anyone around in the mornings where they might see me without a wig. I didn't want to get into any sort of clinch with them where my wig might fall off!

'When I left college I had to find a job and a place to live. I was forced to tell landladies that I wore a wig in case they caught me without it and had a heart attack.

'I was lonely, but I couldn't go back to Wales again and become once more "Mrs Evans's little girl. The one who had lost her hair."'

I was teaching and coping well until a bad bout of flu left me depressed. My doctor sent me to group therapy with a psychiatrist, where I was encouraged to think more of myself and my efforts. I began to see that I had succeeded in spite of my handicap and I saved up to buy my own house.

'I moved in and was happy. Then my previous landlord caught up with me, after his wife died. We got on well. Being my landlord, of course, he has always known about my wig. Harold used to laugh with me about my baldness and call me Gary. That was fine when I was in a good mood but not when I felt low.

'He proposed by saying "You're so busy with the house that you've no time to think about marrying me." I said "All right, I'll give it a try."

At 38, Kathleen married. Her first husband was very tolerant of her baldness. 'He would sit and massage my head, just as my mother had done when I was little. He did say that in the early years he had wondered whether I had been 'up to anything' for such a thing to happen. What could I have done? The mind boggles!

'Baldness didn't matter to him. I could wander around at home without a wig though I did wear a little woolly hat in bed in the winter. We had two years, eight months and eleven days together. He died of lung cancer.'

Two years later Kathleen married for the second time. *'I had to work a lot harder with John and hide my wigs all the time. Still, I understood if he just didn't want to think of me as bald. Every morning I'd be groping about in the bed for my wig before he woke up. It was always slipping off. He hated to see me without a wig and would shout "Oh no, no, no," if he caught sight of me without it, so I changed in the bathroom out of his way. In bed, when I wore the wig, it would often stay on the pillow when I sat up. Very embarrassing.*

'Oddly enough, he was proud of me. He would take me out and whisper "You're the best-looking thing here tonight." He was really pleased when someone told him my "hair" looked nice.'

She was aware of 'pandering' to him. *'I was the sort of wife who tried a little harder. I don't feel quite a "whole woman" with no hair, so I try to please to compensate for it. If he came home in the middle of the night and wanted egg and chips I would get up and make it for him.'*

ROXANNE needs a drink before she can contemplate sex with her husband.

She is tall, her dark bob blends beautifully with her make-up free face. She wears a real hair wig because acrylic wigs irritate her skin. A Londoner, she had a good career in publishing before her marriage. She swings a small boy out of the car and above her head. He is 10 months old, fat, contented and beaming. *'If I hadn't had him I might have kept my hair. Still, I'd much rather have him. I was so thrilled when he was born after two girls.'*

Roxanne lost some hair after every baby was born. Alopecia patches had begun at puberty, cleared up, and then started again at 22 when she was in her first job. *'I was on the pill but don't know if that had anything to do with it.'* It worsened after each pregnancy.

'In my teens, I wouldn't go out with men because of it. I remember during a heatwave, I didn't want to go swimming but a girl friend rang up and said, "Put your scarf on for goodness' sake and come out." She was right. You need someone to give you a shake.

'My first boyfriend hadn't told his parents my terrible secret. (I think that's why we broke up.) He was so embarrassed when he took me home and they realized I was something of a freak.

'My husband had known me for years. We grew up together so he didn't get a shock on our wedding night. Anyway, I was no surprise to him. We'd been living together for ages.

'If I'm in a good mood I can sleep without a scarf or a wig. I've never slept in a wig very much except on holiday where we were sharing accommodation and the other people might have seen me.

'My doctor told me "You have to live with it like a colostomy bag."

'My mother has tried to talk about it. My father has kept up a firm wall of silence. In fact, he managed not to mention it for 14 years. Then, after ages struggling with my own very patchy hair, I came in wearing a wig and he said "There's my girl looking lovely again." He'll never know how much he hurt me. He could accept me in a wig but not as I really am.'

PAULINE lost her hair 16 years ago when her children were small.

'Fortunately,' she says, *'my husband is easy-going . . . he took it well. I've kept my baldness away from everyone all these years. It's been a lonely misery as I've never met anyone else like me. I wear my*

wig as if it were part of me. I don't think people ought to have to see the ugliness of my head, so I keep an old wig to wear at nights with my husband. It's not that I want to lie about my condition. I just don't want to inflict such an unlovely sight on people.'

A big bustling teacher with a grown-up family of sons, Pauline remembers early days with horror. As she talked about it, this large, capable woman began weeping. 'It's just thinking of the awful times — being interviewed by a consultant who lined up some 20 students to peer at my vulnerable head. Then he told me there was nothing he could do. I would just have to learn to live with it.

'When I asked for two new wigs after 18 months' use, the appliances officer lectured me about "making them last longer". I was so smothered in misery in those days that I couldn't stand up for myself.'

Pauline entered full-time teaching as soon as her children were older. 'You have to get yourself out of the house, force yourself into doing something so interesting, so absorbing, that you'll stop thinking "I wonder why that person over there is looking at me like that. Have they realized I'm wearing a wig?"'

Her husband has helped. 'He made me understand that nobody notices as much as we think they do. People might be mildly curious but on the whole they don't give a damn. That person might be wearing false teeth, false nails, or a false bosom. You've got false hair. So what?'

Her pupils have helped too. 'A little boy will come up and remark "Miss, you've got no eyebrows." You know it's just casual curiosity. He'll have forgotten it next minute.

'Close friends are used to it. They just ask "How is it?" occasionally. I say "Oh, much the same. No improvement." We go on to talk about other more important things.'

Pauline brought up her children 'with the daily fear that playful little hands would scalp me in public. Those days are over. I have adjusted. I have learned to live with it as I was told to all those *years ago. I would still like it back because I still feel peculiar. I then felt a freak.'*

HAZEL, *a college lecturer, has had alopecia areata for only a year, unlike Pauline, who has had 16 hairless years to adjust.* 'My husband and children have given me the best help, but other family members seem to be less able to cope.

'Wigs are itchy and uncomfortable. My husband understands this and I wander around the house bald without comment from anyone.

'I frightened the man who delivers our paper one Sunday morning. He nearly had a fit when he saw me without hair!

'My older relations feel sorry for my husband, not me. "Poor Roger. He's got a bald wife", they say. I said to him: "Invite them for Christmas, fine. But don't forget I'll be in the kitchen bald." Acrylic wigs get ruined if you cook in them.'

Whenever possible she goes around 'bald'. Once, playing badminton, she took off her wig in the middle of a game. 'It took the opposing side so much by surprise that their game fell apart and we won the match!

'It shook me when a consultant dermatologist told me I was bald for life. Until then I had been shelving projects "until my hair grows back". Now I have come to terms with my hairless existence and got back to normal.

'My parents and in-laws cannot accept that I am bald. I still get bouts of panic where I would prefer not to go out and yet I've suffered severe claustrophobia for the first time in my life. I hate wearing wigs, I hate "cheating" and yet can only cope with very short periods of being bald in public.'

Hazel's husband is supportive. When he says 'It really doesn't matter', Roger means it. He is not merely saying it to be kind to his wife. 'She lost her hair within two months. It was a shock for all of us, particularly for Hazel. My problem was to make her see that it really didn't make any difference to me. Our relationship is too strong for that.'

He is a business executive, a systems manager. They have two children, aged 3 and 6. 'It hadn't occurred to me that women went bald. I had associated bald heads with weirdos and punks, not with Hazel. It didn't make any difference to me when she lost her hair. Don't get me wrong — I like to see beautiful women — but my relationship with Hazel is more important than that. I said to her "I like to see you in hair occasionally because I miss it. Don't I get an input of choice in this?" I said that for two reasons: (a) because it was true. I do like to see her in hair occasionally; and (b) for the sake of other people in the family. They like to see her looking "normal" and it saves the older ones getting upset, though she has never kidded anyone about the fact that they are wigs. It's quite funny when she takes our son to school and the kids gather round saying "Take your wig off for us." She laughs and does.

'In the summer she likes to go around without wigs because they are so hot, but in the winter a wig at least keeps her head warm.

'The worst moment for her was when the consultant told her she was likely to be bald for life. I'm glad he did. Although it sounded brutal when she was told just like that, I think it was a good thing. She knew exactly where she was and didn't have to mess around wondering when it was going to grow back. She could plan her life properly again.'

They have never suffered from the inexplicable shame which afflicts other sufferers.

'The chaps at work know. They didn't make any big thing of it, just expressed interest and nearly all of them could think of relatives or people they knew of who had suffered from it.

'Hazel's never tried to kid anyone. I hear of women trying to hide it, even wearing wigs in bed. That's just ridiculous. She never needs to do that with me. We now have an even stronger bond.'

CLARE, *the young mother of two, was also surprised when her husband was not repulsed. It had been her biggest fear. 'I thought he wouldn't love me any more. I thought everyone would laugh at me because baldness is a jokey kind of thing.' Clare's husband tries to comfort her. He even applies the prescribed scalp cream to her head every night.*

When her baldness worsened, Clare returned to her family doctor, but a referral to a consultant dermatologist did not help. He told her 'It might come back. It might not.' He had her photographed for research purposes and, when she enquired about NHS help with wigs, explained that the Department of Health had requested doctors to cut down on this kind of prescription, as part of the financial cuts. To qualify, she needed to have suffered from alopecia for at least two years or to be completely bald. Clare still had some hair left. 'You can get some pretty hats these days,' he remarked.

Clare returned home in tears. She raised the money for a wig herself, helped by her mother.

It was at this stage that she started being irritable and taking it out on the children. 'I rang my health visitor. I was so afraid I'd lose control. She said that I must get out of the house and join everything — play groups, coffee mornings, etc. I began to get more confident and decided to tackle my doctor again. Something new and tough came over me. I managed to change my GP and get a referral to another dermatologist.'

This one was more helpful. He said that she was, in fact, entitled to help with wigs and organized it. The new acrylic wigs helped her to feel normal. 'You do your best. You stick on your wig, false eyelashes, pencil in your eyebrows and hope no one notices. No one's actually said anything yet. I've decided that if they are brave enough to ask "Is it a wig?" I must have the guts to tell them.

'My worst moment was at a "wig party" run by a wig manufacturer at a local women's group. People were buying wigs for fun, for fashion! I just sat there in horror waiting for the demonstrator to pick on me, afraid I would have to take off my wig and put another one on! And no one knew I wore one! I had steeled myself with two glasses of sherry before I set out that night, but I learned a lot about making the wigs look nice. I've now bought a very trendy one which has really boosted my confidence.

'Another dicey moment came when my doctor suggested I needed to have my tonsils out. I refused. It was the thought of being in hospital and people seeing me with no hair, in the operating theatre and afterwards in the ward. I made the excuse that I couldn't leave the children.

'The children know. The other day I was changing when my son somehow escaped through the front door and toddled onto the road. He's only a baby and I had to rush out and rescue him because of the traffic. I thought of the motorists seeing me and I didn't worry so much about them seeing me nude as seeing me without a wig!

'My daughter has a toy wig and thinks it's great, just like mummy's. She cried on Christmas Day. She said, "I asked Father Christmas to bring me a bike and mummy some hair, but he forgot to bring your hair."'

The marriage casualties

Clare and Hazel have had the support of their husbands, but not everyone is so lucky.

JANICE's alopecia started in her thirties. A widow, she had married for the second time. This marriage was wrecked, she says, by her second husband's insensitivity. 'He would taunt me in front of other people, say "Look, she's going bald!" I think that was by way of a joke.

'I got so upset about my patchy head that I went to a wig manufacturer where they fixed me up with two hairpieces. They were very expensive and had to be attached at the sides, front and back with *glue. Every time I went to have my hair reset another section of hair was taken up to accommodate the fastening of the piece. The piece was actually clipped into the scalp with a metal clip and it was agony, but I battled on for some years like this. I liked to go to dances with my husband and I hated to see my scalp shining through my thin hair when I looked in mirrors under the spotlights.*

'The hairpiece people were sorry it wasn't very comfortable but they were used to dealing with men and didn't have any female clients. In the end a friend, who happens to be a hairdresser, persuaded me to do away with the hairpieces and cut my hair exceptionally short all over. I felt most uncomfortable and self-conscious for many weeks.

'The hair loss had begun after a hysterectomy at the age of 37. My doctor, going bald himself, said that there was nothing he or anyone else could do. Once the hair had gone it was gone for good.

'Seven and a half years ago my eldest son died suddenly, a terrible blow. I felt I would never recover from the shock and the loss. After this my hair loss became even more apparent.

'My husband's taunts and jokes were only part of the cruel things he used to say to me, often in front of his friends. I began to feel I was going mental. I finally realized I had the remedy in my own hands. When I told him I was starting divorce proceedings, he threatened me with: "I'll make your life a misery and you'll wish you'd never been born. I'll see you end up penniless. You'll be lucky if you even have a candle to keep yourself warm." In spite of his abuse, I knew the divorce wa something I had to go through with. I'd got myself into this marriage and I jolly well had to get myself out of it.

'The hassle and divorce are all over now. I've moved into a new house, I work as a secretary and I feel much happier than I have in years.'

BRENDA *sees her hair loss as a symptom of her unhappy*

marriage. Her hair started to thin when she was in her thirties. She says that she suffered great misery and humiliation through her husband's attitude. After 20 years and four children, she left him and finally divorced him. 'Since then, I've had 10 very happy years. The freedom from stress after the divorce was quite overwhelming. Even my hair improved, much to my surprise. But just when I thought all my troubles were over, the gradual loss started again.'

Brenda thinks it may be due to a hereditary factor. 'I've talked to my own doctor about this and he agrees. It appears to run in my family. My aunt and a young niece both have severe hair loss.'

Now Brenda is facing the problem in her own daughter. From the age of 5, her once-abundant hair has been thinning and now, in her early teens, it is very sparse. 'I've never mentioned my own problem to her,' says Brenda, 'and I've never drawn attention to her sparse hair, but now she's in her teens, looks and hairstyles are so important. And she has noticed for herself. I once heard her weeping in her bedroom and sobbing "Oh, hair!" which cut me to the quick.'

STEPHANIE, a mature student whose marriage ended in divorce after she lost her hair, found her new single state very hard to take.

'Before it happened I had been on top of the world. My husband and I had moved to the North of England from the South-East, both as mature students. I had worked for four years at a South-East college to qualify for a BA (Honours) degree course in design. I was happy and scatty. Then my hair fell out. I was told at the hospital that I had only a five per cent chance of getting it back. I felt terrible, upset and emotionally drained.

'I refused to wear a wig as I felt that was admitting defeat and might prevent my own hair growing back. Gradually I stopped turning up for college. In the end my doctor said I was probably doing myself damage trying to cope with college so I dropped out of the course.

'My husband had gone and I was alone in the house. I didn't go anywhere in case people mocked me. I was new to the city and had no friends. I was scared to go out and only forced myself out of the house so that I could try treatments for my hair. Steroid injections didn't work so I spent money on things like herbalism and hypnosis. I was getting more and more into debt. I was already on the dole but I didn't care.'

A letter arrived from a man she had known in the South-East. He was coming to see her. 'I tried to put him off by explaining the situation but he came anyway. I was panic-stricken. I was so ugly. How could he want me?' Luckily he did. Stephanie has now been living with him for some months. He has a job in a bank, so was able to move north.

And Stephanie's hair has begun to regrow, although a lot is still falling out. 'I don't know whether it is coming or going — both I think! But he is very confident and keeps telling me it will return.'

She is now pregnant. 'My doctor has warned me that I risk losing my hair again after I have the baby, but I can't let my hair problems mess up my life any more. If it goes again, well, it goes! The baby is more important.'

Some women pretend

Some women retreat and hide their baldness even from their families. Some go to extraordinary lengths to keep it a secret.

YVONNE, the wife of a property consultant, lost her hair only a few months after her marriage. She had been a nurse, working long spells of night duty. Doctors could only link her alopecia with exhaustion. Her own opinion is that it may be part of a hormone problem. After her daughter was born she was never able to have another child.

Small, delicately featured, she has shoulder-length blonde 'hair' which makes her one of the most glamorous wives in their set when they go to Ascot or the Derby.

She lives exactly as if she had hair. Every Saturday, she goes off to the hairdresser to have her 'hair' set. Her acrylic wig is washed on her head, rollered, then she sits under the drier alongside all the other clients. They have no idea, she says, that she is bald. 'My hairdresser is very understanding. She does things to a wig which all the manufacturers tell you not to do. She uses heat on it when the wig manufacturers advise strongly against any form of direct heat. But she gets away with it and I always leave the salon feeling absolutely marvellous. My confidence has had a real boost and I feel great.'

She has always felt it wasn't fair on her husband to burden him with the problems of her hair loss. 'After all, we were just married. He had married a young, pretty girl and suddenly she was a bald freak. I couldn't inflict that on him so I've found it much easier over the years to keep my wigs out of his way. If they are in the airing cupboard I move them quickly so that neither my husband or my daughter ever sees them.'

On holiday she even swims in her wig. 'It's amazing how good-tempered the acrylic wigs are. I sleep in them, of course, and it's no problem.

'My husband never mentions it, but being an ex-military man, he likes to see that I look all right if we're going anywhere. At the front door he will check me over and prod the wig if he doesn't like the way I've combed it. Sometimes I feel I'm on parade, but I understand. He married me when I had hair. It wasn't fair on him. We've certainly been very happy for 15 years. Occasionally he comes home and talks about the women he has met during the day — lovely women, apparently. He often remarks on their beautiful hair. I wish he wouldn't. But it's a big part of a woman's appeal, I suppose.'

Some women stay home

HILARY, the industrialist's wife, did not try to hide her baldness from her husband but, as she prefers headscarves to wigs, has often refused to go on business trips with him because she was afraid of the reaction of his colleagues.

'Thirteen years ago my marvellous GP sent me to get a wig. Horror of horrors, I felt like a floosy. From having so little to acquiring this mop they offered me! I preferred my headscarf.'

The fact that she turned up for an interview in a headscarf may have lost her one job she wanted and sometimes she gets comments in the street.

'People will say "Are you selling pegs, love?" One man said, "Haven't you got any hair?" to which I replied, "No, I haven't." You've got to be truthful.'

She spent more than she could afford on travel, searching for a cure, trying everything available. 'I read of a miraculous new primula treatment and travelled regularly to a hospital some miles away for applications of primula leaf to the scalp and systemic steroid injections. For a time, success. I was thrilled to bits with a great deal of hair growth. I even had my hair cut!' But she was putting on weight and worried about the possibility of other side-effects. 'I felt so strange on the steroid injections – I was as high as a kite some of the time.'

Because of her worries, she made the mistake of going against her consultant's advice and stopping the treatment before the end of the course. The result was disastrous. 'We went on holiday to Spain. I was thrilled with my new hair and even swam in the sea. But one day in the shower everything went in one fell swoop. Eyebrows, lashes, pubic hair, underarm hair. I looked like a plucked duck. I shouted to my husband, "I don't believe this."'

The experience was so traumatic it put Hilary off any further efforts to get her hair back. 'I then decided enough was enough. No more injections, no more herbalists, no more trichologists. I would just live and feel much better for it. My body hair has mostly returned, eyebrows and eyelashes too, although one eyebrow lacks colour and still unfortunately no hair on the head.'

Hilary was beginning to feel that she was missing out on trips with her husband. When he was recently sent to Barbados she decided to join him — and purchased two new wigs. It was a wonderful holiday and morale returned.

Some women fight back

SYLVIA, living in West Germany, was terrified of wearing a wig. At 61, she lost her hair during a period of stress. She and her husband were living in Germany for the first time. They had moved there from the UK for the sake of his job. 'I was suffering from nerves when this started. I hated living in a foreign country. Our sex life has been 'no go' for some years. I want to — he doesn't. Then my daughter's marriage broke up. Her husband left her, leaving her with three young children. My doctor seemed to think this all added up to stress which probably caused the hair loss.'

Her small granddaughter came into the bathroom one day and observed, 'Granny, I can see through your head!' Her brother thought that his grandmother looked like a monk.

Sylvia wailed: 'I'm a complete disaster. No social life, no sex life. I'm afraid to go to the door. I look so awful.'

She bought a real hair wig at a cost of £100. 'It's horrible, I wear a cotton scarf all day so that the air can get to my scalp. We're going home to England for Christmas and I'm terrified. They are all kind and loving but my uncle is a shocking leg-puller and is not above teasing me in company. I don't feel I can cope with it.'

Once she had bought an acrylic wig which she really liked, Sylvia survived her socializing without a qualm. 'It's super,' she announced. 'I wore it to a New Year party and felt quite glamorous.

All the family like it too, including the uncle.'

Lately she has had some good news. Her hair is growing back again. Slowly, but it is there.

CAROL *was equally scared of coping with the police ball, but her husband wanted her to accompany him. The wig caused an unexpected stir. 'When we arrived heads turned to look at me. It appeared that some of his colleagues coouldn't believe I was his wife. What they expected I don't know. None of them knows of my condition but maybe the wig creates a different impression. It goes to show that one can still look great with a little effort and a lot of guts. You don't have to hide yourself away!'*

Silence on the subject is the usual embarrassed spin-off from your friends, even your closest family.

WINIFRED, *62, did not tell her husband that she wore a wig when she married, but a year after their wedding he found out. 'The weather was windy. I put my hands to my head to hold the wig on but it was too late. It was such a terrible shock to him that he has never spoken about it to this day.'*

That was nearly 40 years ago.

Survival plan

When a woman loses her hair she sometimes feels that she looks like a man, particularly if she sees a back view of her head in the mirror. I was horrified at first by the horrendous stumpy shape of my skull. I looked like a little old man. The black, hopeless thoughts set in. 'How the hell will any man ever fancy me again? Worse, what if that sympathetic look comes into his eyes?'

You know it's self-pity. You know there are millions

worse off. But you still feel like a man, an ugly bald man.

Make space. Get away for a few days if you can. Give youself time to take stock and evolve your survival plan.

First, take a vow of silence. *Don't* keep talking about it to your partner. He has had a shock too. You have started to cope with it. You are thinking positively – most of the time, anyway – and doing as much as you can to help yourself. You think about hair a great deal, you gaze at heads, bald or otherwise, everywhere you go. But the subject may be a bore or a turn-off for your husband. He didn't marry a baldie, after all. He married you – with hair. Your sudden transformation may shatter him at first, particularly if he is not over-confident himself.

In an ideal world, a life partner should love you for what you really are, not what you look like. But this is not an ideal world and he will need time to adjust. Even if he is not upset, talking about it may bore him, as many men get bored when a woman goes on at great length about her appearance, even if she is a stunning beauty.

So *shut up*. Once you've lost your hair, anyway, there isn't very much to say about it, so restrain yourself from endless moaning. This will have the added bonus of silencing him as well. If he is the type to make jokes – as Kathleen's husband did by calling her 'Gary' (see page 60) – this can be very hard to take. The laughs become a little strained after a while, as she pointed out. She could take it when she was in a good mood but sometimes . . !

You are also going to work hard. When you are lucky enough to have hair you can afford, occasionally, to 'let yourself go', slop around in ancient jeans, wear your face as inno-cent of make-up as you like. But when you have lost your hair, and possibly your eyebrows and eyelashes as well, obvi-ously you are minus an important part of your appearance.

You will have to make up the balance by working harder to look attractive in every other way, every day. Work towards feeling happy about yourself again. Self-esteem and a good self-image are vitally important. No more slopping around for you, no days off. You will adapt your life to your handicap as people adapt when they have more serious medical conditions. The mastectomy patient learns to compensate with a prosthesis instead of a breast. The colostomy patient learns to cope with the inconvenience of a colostomy bag. Our problem doesn't hurt physically. It is not life-threatening. It is, after all, only our hair.

The Worst Thing Is Losing My Eyelashes and Eyebrows. How Can I Look Like a Human Being Again?

Losing these can be harder than losing your hair. Even men have been known to struggle with eyebrow pencils to try to reconstruct the appearance of normality. For a woman it is easier, as people are accustomed to seeing her wearing make-up.

Find an old photograph of yourself to try to match up the eyebrow line. Instead of an eyebrow pencil try a cake eyeliner with a very fine brush to paint in 'hairs' in the direction in which normal eyebrow lines would be going. Yes, it does take ages, but the effect is quite natural. Soft brown is a good colour unless you normally had blue-black eyebrows!

Susan Crabtree, a young college lecturer from Burnley, Lancashire suggests a soft kohl pencil to give the same effect as brush strokes. 'If you don't like the shape you can always rub out the line and start again.'

False eyelashes help, but they need to be the lighter, smaller type, kept mainly to the outer corner of the eye. Taken into the centre, they have the effect of making the eyes look smaller. They should be applied *after* eye shadow.

Susan says she has never found it too much of a problem. 'A perfectly normal look can be achieved by the clever use of eyeliner. Use kohl pencil to draw a line inside the upper and lower lids, then smudge it carefully.'

Without the protection of lashes against dust in the air and particles flying off roads, eyes can get really sore. 'Hypo-allergenic make-up is worth the extra expense,' says Susan. 'Your eyes will also benefit from a good eyebath from time to time, with one of the chemist's soothing eye lotions.'

Don't Put It Off. You Are Going to Buy a Wig. 'Oh no! Has It Come to That? Not a Wig?'

Like me, you will be aghast. 'Only old ladies, judges and drag artistes wear wigs', you will cry, 'not me, a normal twentieth-century woman.' But you will realize, as you start to dread going out in the wind, when you can no longer disguise the bald patches with clever combing, that the time has come to get yourself to the nearest modern wig department.

Faced with rows of severed polystyrene heads sporting coiffures of all kinds, your immediate instinct will be to turn tail. Stay put. I know you think it is the end of the world, as I did. I imagined the discreet postiche parlours of my youth where elderly women, in fur coats, visited the bespoke wigmaker, going *in* with hats strategically placed on thinning hair, coming *out* bewigged – so obviously bewigged, in thick gleaming 'hair-dos' which stood no chance of deceiving anyone. The wigs stood slightly away from their heads at the back, just enough to give the game away.

Of course, I knew about 'fun wigs', a fashion relic of the 1960s, but not a wig to be worn daily! I was terrified.

I was also out of date. Modern acrylic wigs are lightweight and trendy. When you find the right one, you will probably look better than you ever did in your own hair.

Decide first which type you prefer. Some people like the human hair variety, made to measure and costing several hundred pounds. These take some weeks to make and may involve fittings. With a real hair wig, you must also be prepared to spend hours on styling and setting, as it needs to be treated as your own hair. You must not get it wet – that's fun in the British climate! You must also send it back to the manufacturer for regular chemical cleaning.

For me, it was much easier to slip into a department store and buy an acrylic wig 'over the counter'. These have practical advantages. They can be washed at home and, if you are caught in the rain, you need only leave them alone and restrain yourself from touching them until they are dry. Then they are usually as good as new. They are much less expensive than the real hair variety, costing from around £60 and they look amazingly natural.

When you go to buy your wig, ask for a private fitting room. Even the staff cloakroom will do, so long as you are left in peace for half an hour to make your decision. You can't do that properly when surrounded by other shoppers, red in the face with embarrassment and expecting to see your next-door neighbour any minute!

Some women travel miles out of their way to purchase wigs. When I first started Hairline, I was pleased to find a local retail outlet for wigs only a couples of miles away from a new member. I sent her a discount voucher for the store and was amused when she wrote asking for an alternative shop, 30 miles away. As she explained, 'I'm a teacher and I may see my pupils or their parents in the local store.'

If there is no fitting room, explain your situation to the salesgirl who may be able to perform the scarf trick. This is a skilful method of putting on the wig, while shielding your head with the scarf.

If she can't do that, you have an alternative. Wig manufacturers are now setting up postal services. You choose the
style and colour from a catalogue and try on the wig at
home. If you make a mistake, refunds are normally prompt.
And 'wigs by post' come less expensive as the middle man,
the department store, has been cut out.

Don't give up if the first wig you try makes you look like
Danny La Rue in drag. You haven't seen yourself with hair
for a while. Of course it looks like a bush! You *will* find the
right wig. It's a great moment, just like falling in love.

Don't strip it off at night in front of your husband. That is
about as sexy as pulling out your dentures.

FACT: Women Who Have Lost Their Hair are Not Obliged to Take Off Their Wigs in Front of Their Men.

Some women have such a close, confident relationship that
maybe they don't need to worry, but most of us find it easier
to go in for a little strategic deceit, especially at first. A wife
can expect a man to go bald in later life – 90 per cent of men
do – but *he* does not expect to have a hairless wife, ever.

At first, you will probably feel better if you go to bed in a
wig, even if it gets hot and sticky and you end up – like me
– scuttling into the bathroom to take it off in the middle of
the night. You may be saying indignantly: 'Nonsense. I don't
need to hide reality. My husband will love me as I am, whatever I look like.' Fine. Let him see you bald if he is perfectly
happy about it. People must work out what is best for them.

If you are unsure, think first of his sensitivities, secondly
of your own. Do you feel attractive without hair? You do?
Good. Then go to bed with him without your wig. But if you
look in the mirror and think, 'Oh, my God. Something from
outer space!' then you won't turn him on, or yourself.

This is the time to indulge yourself. Treat yourself to a

new dress, splash around the perfume you've been hoarding. Buy yourself as many wigs as you can afford. Don't feel guilty. Think how much you are saving at the hairdresser!

Go into hiding. At least as far as 'getting ready' is concerned. No matter how small your house, you can surely find a quiet corner for major construction jobs. If there is nowhere else, put your wig on in the loo!

Don't leave your wigs lying around. Not only will your family keep falling over them, the police will get a laugh if they come in to sort out a burglary. So put wigs in the cupboard and close the door — now!

There are advantages. You don't need to waste hours under the hairdrier any more, or struggle with rollers. If your holiday plane leaves at dawn, no problem. You will be aboard, complete with a magnificent 'hair-do'. It took you all of five seconds to put it on. After a swim, in your pretty towelling turban, you can put your glamorous hair back on again in the privacy of the changing room.

Before you rush out to be admired in your new wig, do make sure you have put it on properly. It sounds obvious, but it is surprising how many people never really get to like their wigs for the simple reason that they are wearing them backwards! I once spent a morning in the shops wondering why my wig felt uncomfortable. It was on backwards.

It is actually quite an easy mistake to make. I even heard of a hairdresser who put one backwards on a client before she cut it, thereby savaging a wig worth £200, so check that simple detail first. The tapes which are used to adjust the size should be *at the back*. Usually, the manufacturer's label is there too. Place the wig exactly where your hair-line should be, neither too far forward nor too far back.

Wash an acrylic wig at home, in cold water, with a wig shampoo, ordinary shampoo or even washing-up liquid.

Fabric conditioner is a good idea in the final rinse. Officially, wig manufacturers advise us to let the wigs dry naturally away from direct heat, but many people break the rules and get away with it. I have heard of wigs surviving washing machines and spin-driers (on gentle cycle in a pillowcase). Some use electrically heated rollers for setting (on moderate heat). All this is strictly against the advice of the manufacturers. Sometimes a wig salesgirl will offer to wash it for you. This is well worth a tip – a large one.

The wig may slip around like an egg cosy if you have a totally bald head. Wig – or toupee – tape can be purchased very reasonably to keep it still. You stitch the tape inside the wig and you also need an oil silk patch to secure it.

The manufacturers will assure you that the acrylic wigs look just as good after washing. Personally, I disagree as I prefer them new and shining, but some women wash their wigs before wearing them to make them look more natural.

Don't worry if the worst happens and your wig falls off one day. It happens to us all.

NANCY, aged 71, who has been wearing wigs for 30 years, was in a department store with her 2-year-old grandson. 'He was jiggling about and I was trying to keep him fron trampling on my bad foot when I fell backwards. Horror of horrors, my wig dropped off. Where was that hole to fall into? I felt more bothered about my wig than whether I was hurt!'

I was once walking cheerfully through Birmingham, my 'pony tail' bobbing up and down on my shoulders, when a man tapped my arm. I turned huffily, thinking he was making a pass, only to have my alleged 'hair' handed to me. 'I think you dropped this, miss,' he said.

After I had lost my hair completely and was wearing a full

wig, a woman friend was in the garden with me. We were trying to hang out a wet carpet after my washing machine had flooded the kitchen. Suddenly it was caught by a gust of wind and swung back into my face, dislodging the wig. 'How embarrassing!' I groped in the wet grass to retrieve it, with what I hoped was a light laugh. I picked it up and disappeared. I had never told my friend that I wore a wig. Since then, she has never mentioned it and neither have I.

Inititally I fussed a great deal about whether people knew about the little laughs they must be having at my expense, but soon I learned the facts of 'Wig Lore':

- Every time you get out of a car you will catch the wig on the roof. This always happens, especially when you are watched by someone you wish to impress.
- When you are going out on a special occasion, the wig which looked wonderful when you tried it last week will suddenly refuse to comb up. It will not look nearly as good as it did when you tried it on. But remember when you had your own hair? Wasn't it just as difficult sometimes?
- If you go out in a short wig one day and a long one the next, you are bound to meet the same people. Fact of Wig Lore: no hair grows six inches in the night.
- At a party you will not be the only person wearing something false. What about false nails, bosoms, teeth?
- When your hair grows back, you will not throw your wigs away. You will realize how pretty and convenient they were. You will wear them again.
- Wigs bring out the wits. Brace yourself against a world in which there will always be a 'funny uncle' dying to be the comedian of the party at your expense! Let him. The wives will probably be silent and jealous, just wondering where you had your hair done!

4

WHEN IT HAPPENS TO A MAN

'Everything stopped — joy in life, sex drive. It killed
any urge for sex for two years.'

ROSS *is a former army officer. Idealistic, courageous, he has been to war. He has also fought his toughest battle of all, against polio, so baldness should have seemed a triviality. But when all his hair fell out in the space of four weeks, it was a shock which damaged his life dramatically.*

Ross had always enjoyed the company of women. Now, suddenly he didn't want to know. Sex drive vanished as rapidly as the hair on his scalp and body.

He was in his mid-forties. Twenty years earlier he had contracted polio while serving as a young infantry officer in Hong Kong. After fighting in Korea and serving in Japan, the sharp onset of polio put him in an iron lung. At first, doctors expected him to die. Later, they thought he would be paralysed for life. Finally, that he would never again take part in sport. But they reckoned without Ross's determined spirit. 'Of course I'm going to play bloody golf again,' he vowed, and left hospital two years later with nothing worse than a slight limp.

His sudden baldness happened at a time when he had left the army and was a teacher. Confidently male, he was vigorous, cheerful and sexually in his prime, married with three children.

The loss of his hair transformed his appearance. 'I didn't even recognize myself at first. If you want a good disguise, that's the answer. Just shave off all your hair.'

It changed his personality. 'It made him more aggressive,' says his wife.

It changed his life. 'I felt deadened. I wasn't afraid of being unattractive. I don't think I'm vain. I just didn't want sex.'

Women have always indulged him. From the hospital staff who nursed him through polio to the wife and daughters who affectionately boss him around in the large Edwardian house of a university town. Essentially masculine, he speaks in all-male military language. He talks of a 'kip', of 'mates' on the battlefield, of his life in the army, with Sunday morning hangovers and a girl for weekend leave.

Romantic, he writes poetry. Sensuous, he loved the caresses of the nurses and physiotherapists who massaged his muscles back to life when he was ill. Helpless in bed and wheelchair, he thrived on their touch.

Ross, like most men, might have expected to go bald gradually as he grew older, but when it happened so suddenly it was as devastating to him as to a woman. While a wife may feel that her baldness makes her less attractive to her husband, a man who is suddenly deprived of his hair may not worry consciously that it makes him ugly. Ross's reaction was simply to lose interest in the sexual side of his life.

He makes light of it. 'My wife is a down-to-earth Virgo, while I'm a dreaming Pisces. She's very philosophical, I don't think she minded'. But Ross minded a lot, privately.

His ordeal began with a strange purplish rash which appeared on his chest and abdomen. Inflamed, with very dry skin, the rash was sore and painful. Within four weeks, he noticed that his hair was dropping out in thick tufts every time he brushed it. It was July; the school holidays has just begun. He went to the doctor, confident of a cure. 'After all, they had put me back on my feet after polio, so I was sure that such a triviality as hair loss could be easily cleared up. I had childlike faith in medical miracles.' It was not justified. The GP informed him that he knew very little about alopecia and that doctors probably wouldn't be able to cure it.

Ross was referred to the nearest teaching hospital where, as it happened, an international conference of dermatologists was in progress. 'Having had polio, I am used to being a medical guinea pig, so I said I wouldn't mind if the skin specialist looked at me.' Stripped, he stood in a spartan cubicle while five doctors examined the savage rash smothering his skin. His hair had nearly all disappeared to reveal a smooth pink scalp and strangely clammy skin on his body. The medics quizzed him from the superior standpoint of those who were clothed, who had hair. 'What drugs have you been taking?' Does your family have a history of early baldness?' Which came first — the rashes or the hair loss?' He soon realized that they knew no more about it than his GP had done. Ross was despondent. Naked and sore before this group of specialists, he grew angry when one doctor, himself balding, loudly accused him of having venereal disease. Ross had had enough. He decided to do the talking and outlined his theory. He believed that he been poisoned by the chemicals he had been using to spray his garden and which were also in use as weed killers at the school. The doctors were noncommittal. 'You appear to have alopecia areata', was their only comment.

Ross went home, defeated. Pain, frustration, he was used to them, but suddenly he felt as terrified as he had during those frightening days in the iron lung. He was so desperately ill in those days that he has forgotten most of the health professionals who nursed him. He remembers only his physiotherapist. She was big and blonde and her ministrations not only helped him to walk again but also reawakened feelings of sensuality in him. Ross was in love with her. Patiently she manoeuvred him in bed and wheelchair and would come to his bed on quiet nights. He remembers her clearly, though sometimes now he wonders whether it was all hallucination.

But would any woman want him now? He felt exposed to the world, imprisoned yet again in an alien body, as he had been all those years before in that iron lung. This time there was no blonde nymph to soothe him, only the dull ache of depression. He gazed in horror at his mirrored reflection. Who would be turned on by this white 'boiled egg'? Without hair there is nothing to hide behind. A feeling of unease passed through him, like an electric shock. He looked like something from another world. He felt sore, with the rash, and tired. He suddenly felt very ill indeed.

For a man such as Ross, who is sensitive and imaginative, the shock of sudden baldness was a massive blow. For Michael, a graphics artist, it was even more difficult. He had no wife to reassure him.

MICHAEL: *'When a man goes bald in the normal way, gradually, he often looks distinguished. I just looked scruffy.'*

Michael started to lose his hair six years ago at the age of 20. The patches were at the back of his head, one sideburn is now missing and there is a patch at the front. 'It's impossible to cover it all with a hat,' says Michael. 'It won't be long before I lose it all.

'At the time it began I had a rather hectic job in a small printing firm and for much of the time I worked in a darkroom. This made me think that the cause was lack of sunlight, contamination from photographic chemicals, stress — or a combination of all three. I was under pressure at work. At one stage I actually had a bed in the office. But I enjoy being busy.'

His hair gradually regrew, but when his steady girlfriend decided to end their relationsip, it fell out again. 'I don't know whether it was because of my hair that she left me. I wouldn't blame her if it was. My hair was growing back when we were together, but it still looked a bit of a mess.'

When she left him, he began to feel a failure with women. 'I suppose my confidence was undermined. The further hair loss made me even more self-conscious and introverted, though I have always been quiet.' His mother worries about this. 'Michael has always been a quiet boy. One doctor suggested that this hair loss happened because I left him as a child when I had to go into hospital after a miscarriage. Michael was 3 at the time and I left him at home with relations, but I was only away for a week.'

She is also concerned about his lack of social life. 'He should be out meeting people. I would love him to find a woman friend and get married. It isn't right for him to be stuck here with us.' Michael and his parents live in a dramatically beautiful part of the English West Country. His home, an old farmhouse, is very remote. His father works as an accountant in the nearest town. Originally Michael thought he would follow a similar career and took a job as a book-keeper. But he didn't enjoy the work and switched swiftly to art and graphic design.

A dermatologist offered him no treatment and could suggest only wigs, 'but it's harder to wear a wig for a man. Women can have longish sides. I need sideburns and they look terrible when they stand away from the face.' So he wears his wig only occasionally and tries all kinds of potions he sees advertised. He has sampled organic hair restorers, herbs and seaweed, even boiled nettles. 'I now believe in the holistic approach,' says Michael, 'as opposed to treating the symptoms alone. I went to see a local homeopath and so far have become more optimistic through this treatment which involved a complete change of the person, eating habits and so on. You supply all this information to the homeopathic doctor and a composite pill is given to you, relating to your personal needs. I haven't been able to continue as it is too expensive but it has given me new insights into my life – a spiritual understanding if you like.'

He continues to be something of a loner. His mother complains that he makes excuses to 'chicken out' of family occasions such as his cousin's wedding. He has joined a singles' club run by the local *church and found a new girlfriend there — a divorcee, some years older than himself. He was wearing his wig when he met her.*

It took all his nerve to tell her about it, as even going to the singles' club was an effort, 'but I'm glad I did. It has helped my confidence and I'm learning not to take it too seriously. I'm taking constructive steps to get myself out of the house more.'

Isolation and loneliness are faced by many young men when they go bald.

ROBERT *also lost most of his hair through alopecia areata as a child in Canada. At 33, he has never married and has always been too ashamed of his condition even to ask a woman for a date. 'I just know I am a figure of fun and couldn't possibly expect any woman to take me seriously. This thin little body with a wig perched on the top. I get a sixth sense when people are behind me whispering and laughing. In Canada, when I was a child, people were sympathetic. They are more understanding as a nation than the British.' Irritable bowel syndrome has left him severely underweight. He has to put up with daily ridicule in the street.*

Now Robert lives alone in London. His job as a bank executive is demanding and fairly stressful. 'You have to concentrate. One mistake can upset a case for years.' His existence is solitary, broken up only by weekly visits to his mother and one evening a week at a book society.

He decided to take a pen friend, and enjoyed a long corrrespondence with an English girl about 150 miles away. 'We got on famously. Eventually we arranged to meet.' There was only one problem. He had not told her about his wig. 'I worried for ages and decided that I had better break it to her. She wrote back and was marvellous. She said that she didn't mind a bit. 'Everything was fine, I was really excited. But at the last minute she changed her mind. Cold feet, I suppose, though there may have been a genuine reason. Anyway, that was the end of that.'

He has now become accustomed to his isolation. 'Women think I'm peculiar. My wig looks a bit strange. It is real hair, longish, and you would think that with men wearing hair longer these days I would get away with it, but I don't. I'm trying acrylics now in the hope of looking more natural, but they make my scalp itch.

'I started losing my hair when I was seven in Canada. My parents had gone there in the hopes of finding work but it wasn't easy as my father was unskilled. He has always blamed himself for my baldness. He had taken me to a restaurant and I trapped my finger in a glass door, cutting it badly. He took me to hospital where I was given a tetanus injection. Two weeks later, patchy alopecia areata started. It seemed too much of a coincidence to be unrelated to the injection. One dermatologist told me that the vaccination might have oversensitizied my antibodies and caused the hair loss, so my father felt guilty, though I am sure it was just an accident.

'The cost of living was high in Canada and we couldn't afford a specialist, just the local doctor. Nothing could be done for me, he said, so for two years I wore a cap all the time. The teachers and the children at school were quite understanding but when we came back to England I was older and felt my wig was very noticeable.

'In England I went to Great Ormond Street Hospital for Children which, of course, is the best in the world. They put me on systemic steroids but the side-effects were so bad — I put on stones in weight — that they took me off them.'

At comprehensive school in north London he excelled, gaining six O Levels and three A levels. 'I worked hard. I had more faith and optimism in those days.' There was the odd incident at school. The English teacher grabbed my sideburns in the friendly way teachers sometimes grab a handful of boys' hair. He was amazed to find that the sideburns were part of my wig. The whole thing came off in his hand — to the amusement of the class.'

His condition has now deteriorated so much that it is classed as *alopecia universalis. He still attends a hospital skin clinic.*

Robert feels inferior. 'In one of the James Bond books, Ian Fleming described alopecia as "the most hideous disease in the world". I agree, particularly when you lose eyebrows and eyelashes as well as your hair. It robs your face of all its character. I wish I lived on an island entirely populated by people with alopecia. Then I wouldn't have to put up with all the sniggers. I would just look like everyone else.'

ANDREW, *a radio and television salesman lost his hair just before his wedding. He was 24. 'My wife didn't change her mind. She was so busy with all the arrangements that it would have taken a lot more to make her cancel it. But you should see my wedding photographs! I looked a right mess! Morning suit, all the trimmings, the bride in white, and me — in a very poor wig that looked bloody awful. No eyebrows or eyelashes either. What a day!'*

Alopecia areata happened rapidly and within a few weeks he lost all his hair. He faced his wedding night smooth and bald. Scalp and body hair went completely, but his wife was determined not to give him a chance to feel inadequate. 'I thought she wouldn't fancy me. You don't look very macho with no hair. But she was sure it was going to grow back and kept on and on saying so.

'I look at my wedding pictures now and wonder how I could have done it. You have never seen such a terrible wig and I was always messing around with double-sided sticking tape to keep it on. But when it happened I was trainee sales manager for a national chain of television shops. There was no way I could have done that job without a wig.

'My mother had been very ill just before the wedding. I had been living at my mother-in-law's house, sleeping on the sofa, travelling a lot. It was a long way from where I was working. There was mounting pressure at work, worry about sales figures, targets, charts . . . All those things put me under a lot of pressure.'

Andrew feels his wife gave him the most confidence and ensured that their married life did not suffer. 'She made me feel that she wanted me just as much and everything was fine.' They started a family and now have three children, aged 4, 2, and 5 months.

When his hair started to grow back, he held a wig-burning ceremony in the garden, inviting all his friends to join him for a celebratory drink. The hair took two years to regrow, so in the meantime he wore a cap indoors and out.

When his wife went into hospital to have their first baby, he was determined to watch the birth. 'I went into the delivery room wearing my cap. Fortunately the staff were all so busy that no one noticed me, so no one bothered to give me a gown or theatre cap and it wasn't until it was all over that the sister turned to me and laughed, "You've still got your hat on." I laughed as well.'

Sadly, Andrew's pleasure at the return of his hair was short-lived. Seven years later another episode of alopecia occurred and he has now lost three-quarters of his scalp hair again. He was involved in a particularly stressful period at work as a retail manager. 'This time I decided it was time to change my job.'

He now works from home, running his own small business, painting portraits from photographs. 'I have never regretted giving up my selling job. It also means that I don't have to wear a wig this time. I have thankfully dispensed with it and wear a flat cap when we go out.

'It makes a big difference to my life. When I am without hair I really don't want to go out socially.

'I suppose I've treated alopecia as a warning to change my lifestyle. I am much happier now. My hair has started to regrow. It is at the early stage of being "all white" in colour. It just seems slow this time. I'm getting a little anxious.'

Andrew's wife says she was not too alarmed when his hair fell out. 'I had seen alopecia before, in a colleague at work and a friend at church. When my colleague in teaching lost his hair it was usually

when he was overworking or worried, then it would come back. Now
he has retired it is better — very thick and healthy, as he doesn't have
any work to worry about! When it happened to Andrew I felt sure his
hair would come back the same way.

'I didn't even think of cancelling the wedding. He was just as
attractive to me as he had always been, though I know it depressed
him. I just thought how ill and worried he looked at the wedding.
He wasn't so passionate when he had no hair. He didn't want to go
out very much in the evenings.

'When he was managing the shop he used to try to crayon in the
bald patches with black eyebrow pencil. Eventually he gave up and
wore a wig. He was always worrying in case it fell off in the shop or
in a pub.

'When his hair regrew we had a great time! He was turned on
and more loving. We would go out socially again and everything was
fine.

'When it all fell out for the second time he got very depressed. We
stay in most of the time now. I don't mind as I'm pretty tired in the
evenings, having three under-fives to look after. I don't mind so long
as I know this isn't forever. The hair is growing back just a little now
so I hope it will all come back again as it did the first time.

'He feels there are so many things he "doesn't want" to do because
of his hair loss. One important thing I wanted him to do was to have
a vasectomy. He uses his hair loss as an excuse, saying he can't sit in
the doctor's surgery with his cap on! I really don't see that the doctor
will be paying any attention to the top of his head! So I am trying
to persuade him.'

Sometimes, though, there is good news. Hair grows back —
and stays back. Ross was lucky.

ROSS had always impressed on everyone that his hair would return
but first it was very important to him to find out more about the cause.

He was still convinced that both the rashes and the hair loss had been caused by garden chemical sprays. He wrote to the Health and Safety Executive, who interviewed him and made investigations. His dermatologist contacted the various chemicals firms whose products had been in use at his school and which Ross had also used at home. A spokesman for one of the firms acknowledged that some chemicals — the arsenicals — were known to cause 'dermatitis and hair loss', but explained that these were no longer on sale.

The hospital called in a retired dermatologist of some 40 years' experience. He examined Ross and concluded: 'This is probably alopecia areata but I cannot rule out the possibility that it was triggered by exposure to toxic chemicals.'

But Ross still wanted to know the cause. 'I didn't want to sue anyone. The important thing was to try to prevent something like this happening to anyone else.'

Faced with the ordeal of going back to school to cope with the curiosity of young boys, many men would have been tempted to stay at home, but Ross returned to school for the autumn term. Now he was transformed from a hirsute male to this smooth, hairless individual 'from outer space'. Silence fell as he walked into the school library for the first staff meeting of the term. He looked so grotesquely different from the man they had last seen only eight weeks earlier that several colleagues failed to recognize him. Some avoided him completely. One young teacher complimented him on his new short haircut, then fell back in embarrassment when he looked more closely and saw that Ross had no hair at all.

Predictably, the children labelled him Kojak. But their attitude was not unkind. 'To their eternal credit', says Ross, 'not one child ever attempted to poke fun at me.' But they were very keen to have their books marked, prompted by the natural curiosity to take a closer look at his balding head. The school doctor reported that many children had been to see her, usually on some pretext, to enquire about their teacher's health and why he had suddenly lost his hair.

His wife and family supported him. 'I don't think they ever told me some of the comments they heard outside,' he says. 'My wife is not given to hysterics. She was only angry once, as far as I know.' His wife explains: 'A woman acquaintance stopped me in the street with an expression of deep gloom. "How is your poor husband?" she asked and made it quite clear that she thought he was on chemotherapy and likely to die any minute. I told her "He's only lost his hair, for God's sake." When you've been through what we have in our lives — we've lived through wars, don't forget — losing a little bit of hair is nothing.'

It was hardly 'nothing' to her husband. He felt depressed and began to avoid mirrors.

On his next hospital appointment, he was accompanied by his wife. The sister on reception was sympathetic. 'How old is your father?' she asked her. 'I felt about 85,' says Ross, 'a wizened, balding gnome.'

His theory about the garden spray was finally discounted. 'In the end,' says his dermatologist, 'I do not think we were ever able to relate his hair fall to chemical exposure, and it was felt that he had ordinary idiopathic alopecia areata/totalis. Chemicals usually cause hair to fall out in anagen — i.e. their growing phase — whereas alopecia areata gives these rather characteristic clubbed hairs due to the hairs being rushed into their resting/shedding phase. Although various chemicals cause hair fall — particularly cytotoxic drugs used for cancer — there is not, so far as I know, any evidence of this occurring with everyday environmental or agricultural chemicals. A toxic cause was therefore unlikely.'

Ross refused drugs for his alopecia. 'I felt that over the years — with having had polio — my body had had enough chemicals to put up with.' He also refused to wear a wig. 'I was convinced that once I wore a wig my body wouldn't bother go on fighting and replace the natural hair. For the same reason I had always refused calipers when I was recovering from polio.'

Two years after he lost his hair came the first sign of hope. He was in the front of the car, when his young son, in the back seat, spotted tiny hairs on his father's head. Slowly his hair returned. Soon Ross needed to shave again. His body hair, eyebrows and eyelashes came back as well. So did Ross's normal cheerfulness and zest for life. 'It was a great relief,' he admits, 'to discover that normal sex drive can just lie dormant for a while. I felt fine again. It was also a relief to get my hair back again. In spite of all my protests, I had always had a secret fear that it would never return, or come back in a half-hearted way and just look ugly and moth-eaten.'

It is now 11 years since it happened and there has been no sign of a relapse. 'I realized how lucky I was when I heard that only about 20 per cent of patients with total hair loss recover completely. If I had stayed hairless, nothing dramatic would have happened. Life would have gone on as before. It would just have been muted by that strange block which prevented me from being "full of the joys of spring"! When I got my hair back, life started again.'

Survival plan

The young man proudly brushes his thick, plentiful hair. He puts the question confidently to his bride: 'Will you still love me when I'm old? When I'm bald?' He laughs because he knows it won't happen for years.

A man takes it for granted that he will probably lose his hair one day, but *not* that his wife might be a baldie!

FACT: Men are Expected to Go Bald Sometime.

FACT: No Matter How Thick Your Hair is Now, You Could be Bald in a Week — at Any Age — if You Got Alopecia Areata.

FACT: You are Lucky to be a Man. Society Will Accept Your Baldness Easily. If You Suddenly Lose Your Hair, it May be a Shock For You, But it is Not the Freak Happening it Would be for Your Wife.

Having said that, it can still be tough on a man because the effect of alopecia areata is so messy and patchy. If it becomes total and eyebrows and eyelashes also disappear, a man also has a loss of self-image, and feels disbelief – and horror – every time he looks in a mirror.

MARTIN, 17, was a promising sixth-former when he lost all his hair. He excelled in languages, obtained a university place and had hoped for a career in travel.

His hair loss wrecked all that. He lost confidence, was afraid of other people's reactions to him, and gave up his dreams of a career. 'I started to drink heavily which became a problem. I found that women soon left me and I was three times involved in "suicide" attempts – though, as I told someone every time that I had taken an overdose, I suppose they were just "cries for help".'

He took a stopgap job as a betting shop manager and, at 31, finds life very lonely. 'I hide myself away every evening, unless I go to pubs. Where else is there to go? Then the drink problem starts again.'

So how does a man survive it? There are two ways open to you.

You can say 'No one will ever want me without hair. I am going to forget about sex, career ambitions, all the things in life which are important to me, until my hair grows back.'

Fine. Opt out, if you want to surrender before the battle has even begun. But have you considered how long it will take for your hair to regrow? If and when it does grow again, it could be as long as two years before you are anything like your old self.

The alternative is to make the best of yourself as you are. Stop dodging mirrors. Stop denigrating yourself.

FACT: Many Women are Attracted to Bald Men.

How many females have turned down Yul Brynner, Kojak in his prime or one of those sexy, bald pop singers?

Totally bald men are often macho, devastatingly attractive. After all, you have the same body as before. Only your hair is missing.

FACT: Your Wife Probably Won't Give a Damn About Your Loss of Hair.

What will worry her is the effect your hair loss has on you. She may not mind the baldness. She will mind if it wrecks your married life, if you stop taking her out and stop making it fun to stay in. If you call a sudden halt to your sex life, she may not be pleased.

Decide About Wigs

NICK, an RAF sergeant, who lost his hair, found that he liked himself better with no hair at all, rather than the odd scruffy patch. 'I went to many hairdressers but they all refused to shave my head.' Eventually one was persuaded and Nick felt better. 'Once I had no hair at all, I didn't have a problem. I have noticed other people suffering the same way as I do and I must say that they all look very glum, down in the dumps. I now enjoy myself as much as possible. Life is too short. I am what I am.'

Many men feel silly in wigs. Unless a wig is essential for his career, a man is probably better off without one. No matter how expensive, wigs often look a little strange, particularly around the sides. Many men feel happier in cloth caps.

Some feel happiest of all when they have accepted themselves as bald, stopped apologizing . . . and go out with a naked head to let the world think it's deliberate, a new look chosen for fashion. So choose the way that suits you.

Once *you* get to like your new self, the world will follow, I'm certain.

5

WHEN IT HAPPENS TO A CHILD

*'I would mortgage the house — anything — if I
could get my daughter's hair back!'*

When a child loses hair suddenly, the situation is often as traumatic for the parent as for the child.

It is estimated that, of all patients with alopecia areata, 40 per cent of males and 31 per cent of females develop it before they are 15.[15] Among children who lose all scalp hair, 21 per cent show no significant regrowth and only 1 per cent achieve permanent regrowth, according to American research.[16] But, more optimistically, 44 per cent of the children who develop total hair loss have subsequent significant periods of normal/near normal hair growth.

ADAM was 18 months old when it began with a small patch on the crown, then another. His grandfather has always suffered from AA and was 90 per cent bald at 14. He says: 'I don't want Adam to face the teasing I had from other children.'

Alopecia's effect on children can be horrendous as they grow older.

PEPPI, aged 13, slashed her arms with a penknife in the playground of her comprehensive school. Her mother says: 'Peppi did it out of sheer frustration. That day I realized just what an effect the loss of her hair had had on her. I made a fuss and demanded that the headmaster and our doctor call in a child psychiatrist.'

It is now two years since Peppi lost her hair totally, including eyebrows and eyelashes. The family still reels from the shock. Her mother describes it as a nightmare for the entire household. 'I wake up every morning with this strange sense of grieving. I would mortage everything if I could only get Peppi's hair back.'

Peppi's parents have worked hard to achieve their present comfortable lifestyle. Their detached house is the biggest in the suburban London crescent. Her father is a successful manufacturer of office equipment. He is stunned by the extent of his daughter's condition and the fact that no amount of money can help her. 'If only doctors would tell you the truth from the start,' he says. 'We were told that it was only a minor disorder and would soon clear up. Now it looks as if it could go on for years.'

Peppi's problem began at 11. Her cousin, a hairdresser, was perming her hair as a special treat. Peppi had been playing with a glitter spray, the kind which gives hair gold and silver sparkle. Her cousin joked: 'Look, your hair's gone green!' She looked more closely and stopped joking. There were several small bald patches all over the child's head. Two weeks later, Peppi was completely bald. Menstruation began around the same time.

Having an idea that it might have been caused by stress, her mother put it down to an incident a few weeks earlier. Her older sister had taken Peppi to play with a group of other children. They went to the shops and the others got involved in shoplifting. 'It was done only in play but they had a ticking off from the police. It must have upset Peppi more than we realized. She was only an onlooker but perhaps she felt guilty.'

As in many cases where a child has lost hair severely, it is the mother who seems to suffer most. 'I get very withdrawn. It is awful to see a child who has been normal and happy suddenly changing. She is aggressive now, much too loud. When she lost her hair, the little girl who played with dolls disappeared and this big noisy teenager came in her place. She seems to behave like this to make up for her lack of hair.'

Peppi is tall, womanly before her time. Wearing her trendy new blond wig, she can easily be mistaken for an 18-year-old. It has all made her mother over-protective. On windy days, she keeps Peppi away from school. Often she meets her in the car at tea-time.

'When she tore her arms I thought she had exploded at last after all the teasing she gets at school. The children give her hell, particularly the older boys. They try to drench her wig with water. It is a new one, supplied by the hospital, and they seem to try to make it look a mess. Sometimes they throw balls at it in the playground. She was looking forward to going to a disco but a gang from school waited there with a camera poised to take her picture as they knocked her wig off. The kids' cruelty is unbelievable.'

When it first happened, Peppi was not keen on wearing a wig. She preferred to wear caps, indoors and out. 'One cap fell off in the street and blew away. But luckily I was with her so I put my coat around her head and shoulders and rescued the cap. It made us finally decide she must have a wig so we went to the hospital to see about it. But it caused problems on holiday when it fell in the sea.' Her sisters, swimming with her, managed to get the wig back in place before they came out to face the crowded beach.

Medical treatment with systemic steroids failed. There was no regrowth but Peppi put on a stone in weight. The family also spent a considerable amount on homeopathic treatment without success. Peppi also suffers from eczema and asthma.

The family has no previous history of alopecia, though they are fairly hair-conscious. Peppi's father recently had a hair transplant although his problem is just male pattern baldness.

Her mother tried to compensate by buying Peppi plenty of lovely clothes. 'It's all I can do. I spend a fortune.'

When a child is in the public eye, coping with alopecia can be even more difficult for a parent.

TONI *Warne was only nine when she became a television star after winning BBC TV's Bob Says 'Opportunity Knocks'. She had had alopecia areata since she was two. Patches had come and gone, growing back each time.*

Although the latest patch was growing in when she won the TV contest, her mother says: 'I still had a job to disguise it under the spotlights. So I had her hair cut and lightly permed. Reporters asked me whether I was trying to make her look like Shirley Temple so I had to explain to them about her alopecia. Some people, who read it in the papers, asked whether she was under stress because of so much TV work but, in fact, her hair has been a lot better since she started on TV. She really loves singing.

'I used to cry over it when I washed her hair and saw the bald patches. The doctor warned me not to let her see that I was upset. He said that it was bad for her to know how worried I've been.

'I was also told not to spoil her, which I was doing – to compensate for the baldness, I suppose.'

Toni finds that the natural jealousy of her peers comes to the fore when they see her in the street. She says; 'Other children shout "Baldie" or "She's on the telly and she's bald!" It used to upset me but now I realize that they are just jealous. The trouble is that in the swimming pool my hair gets wet and they can see the patches.'

Her hair is improving. From having four patches she now has only one, so her parents are optimistic.

JOANNE went bald at seven, and her parents were surprised by the lack of help they received. She had a year's treatment from a consultant dermatologist, using steroid creams applied to the scalp and a minoxidil solution, without success. No further appointments were made. Her parents were told: 'There is nothing more we can do.'

Says her mother: *'I just couldn't believe it. The child had lost nearly every hair on her head and all they could tell us was that she must wear a wig. She won't. She hates wigs.'*

At seven, Joanne was barely out of babyhood, but there was no way her mother could persuade her to change her mind. She regarded wigs as a hot, sticky nuisance and invariably pulled them off. *'There was nothing more the hospital could suggest. I came out feeling we had been turned away and I was just being left to get on with it by myself.'*

Soon, Joanne, who had had long curly hair, took to wearing only shorts and T-shirts which matched her boyish head. She has only a small growth of hair at the nape of her neck. *'She used to love party dresses, ribbons and frills. Now she won't have a dress on her back,'* said her mother.

At school, it was reported that Joanne had been seen using the boys' toilet. The school doctor suggested she saw a psychiatrist. Joanne's mother was furious. *'She doesn't need a psychiatrist and I don't believe she went into the boys' playground. I'm having lots of talks with her and I'm sure it's just a stage she's been going through. She is beginning to be persuaded to put on dresses again.'*

She feels guilty about her own long blonde hair. *'I feel so awful seeing Joanne like this. It hurts to see her. I'd gladly give her all my hair if I could.'*

Joanne won't talk about her loss of hair, except to report the behaviour of a visiting netball team. Unlike Joanne's friends at the village school, they had not known her before her hair loss and had not been able to see what happened. Surprised by her baldness, they behaved very badly. *'They treated me as a joke,'* says Joanne. *'They pointed at me and called me a boiled egg.'* If Joanne was hurt, she didn't show it but merely wandered off into another playground.

Her mother says this is typical. *'She never shows how much she is upset by people staring at her in the street and making silly remarks, but deep down inside I know she feels it. All the visits to doctors, the poking and prying. You can't go through all that without suffering.*

'We don't know the cause. It has been suggested that it was something to do with her grandfather's sudden death. She was very close
to him and very upset when he died. I have never known a child cry
so much, all night. At seven, it obviously hit her hard.'

A few weeks later, her mother noticed long strands of hair on
Joanne's pillow. She touched the hair and great tufts came out easily
from the roots. It went very quickly, leaving only a small section at
the back.

For her parents, in their tiny fishing village, it is a strange sensa-
tion that something 'odd' has happened to their daughter. They find
it helps to enlist the support of the local community. 'No child at the
village school has ever been nasty, mainly because the children saw it
happen, how the hair fell out over a few weeks. They knew her when
she had a normal head of hair like theirs. It is only strangers in the
village who make life unpleasant.'

LAURA's father was very angry when he accompanied his wife and
daughter to see a consultant dermatologist. Laura had started to lose
her hair in tiny bald patches when only a few months old, but the
worst deterioration happened at puberty, when she was 13. She lost
all her hair.

Her father was horrified by the attitude of the consultant. 'He
glanced cursorily at her scalp and offered us nothing. I demanded to
see an alternative consultant but he was no better. All she has ever
been prescribed is a tube of cortisone scalp cream. What alarmed me
more than anything was the lack of counselling. No one could give
us any help in coping with the psychological problems faced by an
attractive teenage girl when she loses all her hair.'

In spite of her parents' efforts to persuade her into a wig, Laura
still wears it only occasionally. She is quiet, hardworking, very much
an achiever. She is also something of a worrier. She says: 'That year
when I lost my hair completely — when I was 13 — is just a year

blacked out of my life. I couldn't cope with a life in which I was completely without hair'. Her brother and sister have been teased at school about it. Some youngsters suggested that she had shaved her head deliberately in a 'punk' style.

Children – the doctor's dilemma

Laura's is a familiar story. Baffled parents find that the hardest thing to take about alopecia in a child is the bewildering silence on the part of some doctors. Often kind and always polite, doctors may be deliberately noncommittal. One reason for this could be that the prognosis, especially when alopecia happens in a child before puberty, is not hopeful.

Research in Chicago which followed up patients over 20 years found that of those developing alopecia areata before puberty 50 per cent became totally bald and none recovered.[17] But if the child was older – i.e. after puberty – the chances of regrowth were more hopeful: only 25 per cent of those developing alopecia areata after puberty became totally bald, and 5.3 per cent recovered completely.

As mentioned earlier, rather depressing statistics emerged from American research which found that only 1 per cent of children with total hair loss showed complete regrowth, but 44 per cent of these developed periods of normal or near-normal regrowth.[18]

In Pennsylvania, a study of 50 patients with alopecia universalis (total hair loss of scalp and body hair) showed complete recovery in only 20 per cent of patients of all ages, with a worse prognosis if it started in childhood before puberty.[19]

'If the child is atopic (suffers from eczema or asthma as a family trait) and loses hair totally before puberty, it is unlikely to regrow permanently,' says Dr Rodney Dawber, consultant dermatologist, Oxford.

When alopecia begins in childhood, it often runs quite a lengthy course of up to 10 years, according to Japanese research.[20] The progress of alopecia areata is so eccentric, however, that it is quite possible the hair will regrow at any stage, even many years after the attack.

'It's important to tell parents that anything can happen in terms of regrowth,' says Dr Dawber. 'We do not want to tell them that the prognosis is bad for their child. If we predicted that the hair would never return, it is quite possible that we could be proved wrong.'

Some specialists prefer not to give treatment to a child. 'I feel that it is quite wrong to inflict the discomfort of such things as scalp injections on a child,' says Dr Andrew Messenger, consultant dermatologist at the Royal Hallamshire Hospital, Sheffield. 'Some patients – and parents – can tolerate having no physical treatment. Others can't.'

Does Alopecia Areata Run in Families?
Family history is important, say dermatologists, as it influences whether you have a predisposition to organ-specific auto-immune reactions, the atopic state or emotional stress.

A positive family history of alopecia areata has been found in betweeen 20 and 27 per cent of cases. About a fifth of patients with alopecia areata can recall a family member suffering the same problem, but it is not a hereditary condition – there is nothing to say that it will definitely be passed on, so *no justification* for saying, 'I will not have children in case they get alopecia.' They might; they might not. The chances are, they won't!

When You Lose Your Hair in Childhood, What Are the Long-Term Psychological Effects?

If losing your hair makes you feel 'different' from other children, this can have a lasting effect.

PATRICIA *was 13 when her alopecia began, at puberty. She is now 33. 'Our family doctor, trying to be kind, said it wouldn't spoil my beauty. He told me to go away and forget about it. But I lost most of my hair as the disease progressed. Looking back, I feel I should have been given far more help but in those days I knew no better. My parents were well meaning but it was all talked about in whispers.*

'When it became really serious and practically all my hair had gone, the dermatologist gave me special shampoos but they made no difference. Heat treatment helped for a while but when that stopped so did the hair growth. The hospital discharged me but promised to get in touch "if any new developments would help". I never heard from them.

'School was horrific. Everyone was so polite and didn't mention it. I found the silence harder to cope with. If only someone had talked to me about it! If I'm honest I suppose that's the reason I left school at 16 instead of sitting A levels.'

She went into an office job and began to make relationships. 'I found that young men accepted me as I was without question. I wasn't as terrible as I had imagined.'

She is now married and has two children, both profoundly deaf. 'I suppose the worry about the problems they will have to face in life has put my loss of hair into perspective. I've now been without hair longer than with it and you do adjust. A sixth sense builds up inside you, making you wary of dangerous situations like windy days in public places!'

KATHLEEN, *who has had alopecia universalis for 45 years,* *remembers growing up with patchy hair loss in a little Welsh village. Ultraviolet light — sunshine therapy — was used at Cardiff Hospital and her mother would massage her scalp every night. At six, her hair grew back, thick and strong. In the meantine, her mother disguised the bald patches with clever hair-styling.*

But family life became fraught. Her sister was locked in perma-nent conflict with her father because she didn't want to go to univer-sity. 'My father obviously got depressed because he hadn't had the chances we had, being a miner all his life. They were both extroverts. They could shout and thoroughly enjoy their quarrels whereas it just depressed me.'

At 15, the problem recurred with one large patch merging into others. 'I would sit playing with my hair and it would come out in masses. My mother was so distressed that she threatened to kill herself if it all fell out.' In six months it had all gone.

'As I had suffered before we knew the ropes but this was wartime, 1942, and so it wasn't of much significance. I had spirit soaps and rubs as well as the ultraviolet treatment. Someone suggested rubbing my head with whisky and castor oil. I hate whisky to this day!

'The neighbours looked at me askance. I was going into the sixth form at school so my mother asked the consultant whether I could wear a wig. He agreed. He said it wouldn't stop my hair from growing.

'My first wig cost 13 guineas at a time when my father was earning £4 a week. The chapel people offered to start a fund but this was "charity" and my mother wouldn't hear of it. Some neighbours did help us, however, and we saved as well.'

Before she returned to her studies wearing the wig, her mother took her on holiday to stay with her uncle in Essex. 'I wore the wig and it seemed such a thatch, such a lot of hair! I couldn't get my hat on top very well and in those days a hat was essential. I rammed on my "Deanna Durbin" — big brim and all! It balanced on top of this great haystack. But when we arrived my uncle greeted me with

"What lovely hair, just like your uncle!" which pleased me. All the cousins complimented me on my "hair" and that went some way to restoring my confidence.'

Back at home, though, the small Welsh community was not particularly kind. 'The boy next door had been home on leave from the army. His mother told me that he had described me as "that girl with all the hair". They seemed to delight in putting me down.

'The wig fell off in the village street. No wonder. It was like an egg cosy balanced on a boiled egg. No one had told me that it would need cleaning. I wore it for three years without cleaning and when it rotted I sewed it up again.'

At her teacher training college, gym was part of the curriculum. 'One of my bleakest moments was when we had to stand on our heads. My wig fell off and all the domestic staff laughed.

'I also needed to wear make-up with the wig to make it look right. My first eyebrows were a mixture of vaseline and soot applied with my little finger. I also wore lipstick, to the horror of my teachers. Make-up was strictly forbidden.

'I was soon in trouble and ended up in floods of tears in the deputy head's room. There was little sympathy. They were straight-backed spinster teachers, apparently afraid to show any humanity.

'I poured my heart out to the deputy head but after that no one ever mentioned my lack of hair. A dreadful silence had fallen over the subject. It must have irritated them that I had three mornings off every week for hospital treatment, not only untraviolet but a rather painful process in which they blistered the skin and tufts of hair grew back in the affected areas. But they soon fell out again.

'When I was 24 I decided to call a halt to the treatment as the travelling was expensive and it didn't seem very successful. My mother didn't want me to give up hope of my hair regrowing but I explained how I felt to the hospital consultant. He did something very clever. He gave me my notes to take to my GP, obviously knowing I would read them. They said "continue the treatment for *the satisfaction of the patient." I knew then that it was hopeless and my hair would never return.'*

Kathleen was forced to come to terms with it. *'One had children calling out in the street: "Hey girl! Are you bald?" But I was, so there was no point in denying it. On open day I was interviewing parents and my mother happened to be visiting me. A waiting parent said to her "Look at your daughter. She's just like a painted doll."*

'Another time my stepdaughter-in-law was complaining that she was losing her hair after having a baby. I felt she was worrying unnecessarily but my sister interjected "You must remember, a woman's hair is important to her." That left me more shaken than any other comment. I may be a widow but according to her I wasn't even a woman.'

A lifetime without hair has had its effects. She remembers as a child she was too shy to ask for sweets in a shop because she thought people would laugh at her. *'What has it all made me? A fighter, I suppose. I'm regarded as friendly, outgoing, poised . . . but at heart I'm still that shy, retiring little girl who was afraid to ask for sweets in the shop.*

'I'm still suffering but, by gum, they are not going to get me down. I don't have any dirty disease. I have my own teeth. My illness is not of my own making. But I've yet to find a doctor who is sympathetic to the emotional traumas.'

Survival plan

FACT: It is Far Worse For You Than it is For the Child. You fear for your child's hairless future. You envisage the problems it may trigger in relationships. But your child is only concerned with today.

- Treat it as a normal ailment, as commonplace as measles or chickenpox.
- Call it by its proper name. It is not a 'deformity', a 'handicap' or even an 'illness', neither is it anything to be ashamed of. It is a scalp disease.
- Discuss it. *Please* don't go silent on the child. Explain that this is a disease which can affect anyone.

Luckily alopecia doesn't hurt; the child will not have to stay at home from school and will be able to do everything normally. Emphasize that swimming, sports of all kinds, can still be enjoyed. Swimming may be even improved. Some people deliberately shave off all their hair because they think they can move faster in the water. If the child is embarrassed, there are swimming caps. Towelling turbans, on sale at many chemists, are ideal. If she is extrovert enough, your daughter could wear one of those swim hats with big plastic flowers.

The child needs a friend, a confidant. It may be a parent, a friend at school or a teacher, but it is essential that there is one person with whom the problem can be discussed.

Brothers and sisters may help. Supply them with the facts on alopecia. They may help you by fending off ignorant comments.

The excuse: 'I can't do it because of my hair' must be banned from your house. Normality is the key word. Don't give the child the impression that something strange has happened. The silence surrounding the subject convinced me long ago that I was not only bald but bonkers, and I was grown up. How do you think a child feels?

If *you* can't cope with it – if it makes you feel guilty, insecure, threatened, to see your child without hair – for goodness' sake don't let that feeling rub off on to the child. Don't make it into a tragedy. The mother who weeps when she sees her daughter's bald patches must make sure she weeps alone, not in front of the child.

Be positive. There is always the chance that it may get better. But to get the hair back must not become the be-all and end-all. Concentrate on improving the quality of life *now*. Cope with baldness by finding out as much as you can about the condition and get hold of all the modern aids which will help, the wigs, the sticky tape, the attractive clothes which will compensate and divert attention to another aspect of appearance, until you are coping as a family and living with the problem.

When, together, you have done all you can, the hair may well grow back and it will be a bonus. But if it doesn't you will have learned to live without it.

Don't go to war with the dermatologists. They may seem to be 'playing the big doctor', being busy, dismissive, brusque. They may feel anxious and guilty about offering so little help. All they have to offer are treatments which rarely work on a condition which may or may not get better by itself. No wonder they feel demoralized! Unfortunately, they may go for a bland 'It's bound to clear up soon' attitude, simply because they feel so inadequate.

There is a need for some kind of counselling for families – a counsellor who could help sort out the best ways of coping with this condition. Families feel rejected by the medics, sent home to cope alone with a condition they do not understand. More information, more talk, should come from a counsellor, perhaps attached to the school. It doesn't need to be a psychiatrist. The 'stigma' of seeing a 'shrink' often upsets people more than having *no* advice.

Help the child to see the situation as an advantage over other children. No boring sessions at the hairdressers, no arguing with parents about getting hair cut. Your child can have hair that looks smart any time the wig comes out of the cupboard. Talking about it sensibly with other children may help. A few 'fun' wigs may raise a laugh. If the child can smile about it, you could be winning.

When It Comes to a Wig

Dermatologists emphasize the importance of persuading a girl to wear one. Apart from improving her appearance, she needs one to keep her head warm in winter and protect her skull from bumps. It will help her feel normal. Anything which makes her different from the others at school – even a cardigan button – upsets a child.

Indulge a little girl with wigs. Make the outing to the shop a treat and give it plenty of time. Let her choose the one which she likes, even if it is a totally impractical Cinderella job. Let her have it. She will come round to the more convenient short styles later. Make wigs *fun*. Let her try on as many as she likes. The main thing is for her to be happy about it.

Above all, don't put on your uptight tragic face in the shop. Save your 'How could this tragedy have befallen my lovely daughter?' face for when you are away from her.

For field games, cater for windy days by sewing double-sided tape inside the wig to anchor it.

If the child refuses to wear a wig, don't force the issue. Try a little friendly persuasion, appealing to the child's good nature. Explain that a wig is a good idea for the sake of other people's sensitivities. 'You don't want to upset grandma' may work with an older child.

But if the child is really dead set against it, you can't insist. After all, who is she wearing the wig for? Herself or you? Because you want to see your pretty daughter looking glamorous again with 'pretend' hair? If she doesn't see it that way, it is on her own head, not yours. With a bit of luck, she might be persuaded to wear a trendy baseball cap as a compromise.

Best of all, introduce her to another child who has lost her hair, if possible. This is something parents often arrange through Hairline, and it works brilliantly. Children, as well as adults, like to know that they are not alone and that there are others in a similar situation.

6

WHEN IT HAPPENS TO THOSE WHO ARE SINGLE

'I realized that life is too short to waste worrying about a bit of hair. I set out to win.'

'What's your problem, Dunc?' The question came from an old friend, a chap Duncan Goodhew had known all his life.

Champion swimmer, Olympic gold medallist, Duncan Goodhew is world-famous. At 36, he is a success, but he says: 'If that old mate of mine hadn't asked me that question I might still be sitting at home, moaning because I'd got no hair!'

At the time Duncan was 16. 'I was very depressed, sorry for myself. I felt that I was a total flop. Without hair. Without hope.'

He lost his hair at the age of 10. Alopecia universalis followed a bad fall from a tree. His hair has never regrown.

'In my teens, I had given up hope of getting my hair back. It was a difficult age to lose your hair, when everything depends on your looks, meeting girls and so on. So I apologized all the time. When I met a new girl I would say, "Hello, I'm Dunc. I'm sorry I'm bald." Naturally nobody wanted me.

'Then came that question from my old mate. I saw the quizzical look in his eyes and knew at once what he was thinking. He was a cripple. He'd had a lot of illness all his life. Compared with him and what he'd been through, my loss of hair was nothing! From that moment I stopped saying sorry.

'I might never have made anything of my life, certainly wouldn't have got to the top in sport, if it hadn't been for my old friend and that change of outlook.'

At school in Sussex, he suddenly became the comedian of the class. He would wear a long wig and wait for some visiting master to tell him to 'Get your hair cut, lad.' Then he would whip it off and have the class falling about with laughter. As his popularity grew, girls came along naturally. On the street he would doff his wig to them, like a hat. Duncan was a joke, a good sport. He convinced them that he didn't mind being bald. He laughed. The world loved him.

'When it first happened, I'd been hit for six. I went everywhere for treatment, tried all sorts of quacks, let doctors put all kinds of lotions on my head. For years I just lived for the day when my hair would grow back. But it didn't, and after I changed my attitude I didn't care whether it did or not.

'Everywhere I go we have a laugh about it. Kids tease me and I say to them, "You've got a lot of hair. Can I have some?"

'People think it may have helped me with the swimming — they reckon that being bald helped me to swim faster. I'm not sure about that. What happened to my mind and approach to life was what mattered. Adversity either makes or breaks.'

He is now married. His baldness has never bothered his wife. 'Think how lucky I am. At my age, most men are worrying in front of the mirror that their hair is receding. I've got the worst over. I'm lucky.'

If losing your hair when you are married brings its problems, to go bald when you are single can be even more traumatic. The letters that pour in to me from single people say it all:

- 'I am desperately worried. It's turning me into an agoraphobic, never wanting to go out' — from a 27-year-old girl student.

- 'I get so very, very depressed because I don't have all my hair. I sometimes want to die because of it. It's an unfair and cruel disease. I hate the word "bald"' – from a 19-year-old, losing hair in patches.
- 'I come back to my flat here in Monte Carlo and take off my wig. Living alone, I can walk around at home without covering my head. It stops me thinking of getting married. A husband might find me unacceptable, unattractive' – career woman, early forties, working in Monaco.

When you are losing your hair and you are single, it can ruin both your career and your hope of stable relationships.

'These are the people I worry about,' says consultant dermatologist Dr Andrew Messenger. 'The single patients who have lost their hair are the ones to keep an eye on. It has happened at a stage in their lives when they are most vulnerable. You must talk to them, watch out for the potential suicide.'

JANE went to a disco with her boyfriend on Christmas Eve. She was 18 and had been losing her hair for two years. That night she struggled very hard to disguise her bald patches with a scarf, but it was difficult. The taxi arrived before she had even put on her make-up . . . the evening started badly.

At the disco, a row developed with her boyfriend. His ex-girlfriend turned up. Jane felt she couldn't compete with the other girl. With her balding head, she felt a mess. She drank more than usual and took some antibiotics she had been prescribed for influenza. When she arrived home in tears, the family had gone to bed. Jane spotted her mother's sleeping pills on the sideboard and took them all.

Her mother says, 'It was touch and go. All night at the hospital we thought she was going to die. She had never come to terms with losing her hair, and her boy's rejection of her made her try to kill herself.'

Jane is a hotel receptionist. She says: 'For months my patches had been getting worse, so that my woman boss at the hotel used to try to comb it up for me to hide the baldness. My boyfriend was threatening to finish with me. I thought that if he left me, who would want a girl with no hair?

'After taking the overdose I realized what I'd done and panicked. I woke up the household. But I was getting sleepy and my brother poked his fingers down my throat, trying to make me sick, saying: "How could you do this to me?"

'Afterwards I realized I'd got to pull myself together and went to get a wig. I bought a most expensive real hair job because I thought it would be best . . . but it was dreadful. It looked just like a busby so I went to our local store and found an acrylic. It was long and curly. I went out that evening wearing it, but my boyfriend didn't seem to like it. We had an awful evening. I came home and cried again. But the next day he said "I quite like it actually".'

Jane is married now and pregnant. Her hair has not improved. She says 'I manage. I take off the wig at night — I'd be too hot trying to sleep in it — and I put out the light quickly so that he doesn't see me!'

GIUSEPPE's father came to wake him to work in the fields of their farm near Naples, Italy, but he found his son dead. He had taken a cocktail of garden poisons and arsenic.

Giuseppe, 17, had left a note. 'Sorry, Dad . . . I've poisoned myself. I can't bear to live without hair on my head because that means no girls and no wife.'

His father said: 'He spent all his money on lotions — even "miracle" potions — to try to make his hair grow.'

Being bald too young can also wreck your job opportunities.

BECKY, *working in a Buckinghamshire supermarket, grew tired of wearing her wig.* 'It used to itch on a warm day so I started to go to work without it, but the manager told me I would be taken off the checkout immediately if I didn't put it back on. I don't know why. The customers didn't mind. In fact, one woman, shopping with her four-year-old, was delighted because her little boy had alopecia as well. She wanted to show him that he wasn't the only one!'

SUSAN *had a lifelong ambition to join the police. When she was about to leave school, she enquired about the possibilities of joining her local force. She was visited by a woman police inspector.*

'I explained that I wore a wig because I had total alopecia, and I was told that I wouldn't have a chance of joining the force. The woman explained that I might be involved in scuffles — it was a tough life — and there was a danger I might lose my wig. I was so embarrassed and miserable, I didn't take my job application any further.'

Giving up hope of joining the police, Susan took a job in commerce. She wore her wig all the time.

'But one day I was in the cloakroom brushing it — I still had it on, I was just brushing it normally — when a woman colleague commented "Your hair must be tough!" So I confessed that it was a wig. The next day my boss called me in. He said "We've heard you suffer from alopecia. That's a nervous condition, isn't it, so you are probably unstable."

'That was it. I had to go. These days perhaps I would have fought back, taken it to a tribunal or something. But they were so horrible, so ignorant, I just ran away.'

Susan went to work for the social services department. 'They were fine, no problem, but I keep my wig on all the time. I don't think it's fair to my clients to go without it.'

LESLEY: 'Every Sunday when I climb into the pulpit, I hope my wig won't slip in front of the entire congregation!'

It was the greatest day of Lesley's life. She was among the first group of Church of England deaconesses to be ordained. The church hierarchy had finally relented and allowed women to take holy orders.

The cathedral was packed with press, TV cameras, relatives, church dignitaries. Lesley knelt before the Bishop. He put his hands on her head in blessing.

'I was terrified,' says Lesley. 'In the middle of that great, awe-inspiring service, I thought "Oh please, don't let him knock my wig off."'

Lesley's career in the church is vitally important to her, but she only made the decision to apply for training after years of agonizing. 'It was fear of being in the public eye. Everyone is looking at you as soon as you step into a pulpit.'

Lesley's hair loss began at 16. At first, she suffered the patchy baldness of alopecia areata but now, at 34, she has lost most of her scalp and body hair.

'I was working in a religious publishing house. I felt I had a call to enter the church but I hesitated for a long time. Losing my hair has made me feel an oddity. It sets you apart from people.'

Lesley was aware that she was allowing her hair problem to put her career in jeopardy and prevent her from taking up work which she knew was right for her. But was she the right person to enter the church, distracted as she was by the problem of her baldness? 'I asked two very close friends to go away and pray. "They must make my decision for me", I'd decided. They returned a few days later and, separately, gave me the same advice: 'Your gift is for people and parish life. Use it.'''

On her application form she had to admit to both poor eyesight and alopecia. 'I dreaded the interview board, but the doctor was very understanding and only referred to my hair as "your problem" so I wasn't embarrassed.'

When she started work in a church, she was wearing a hand-

made, real human hair wig. 'I looked a bit frumpish but I couldn't change wigs in case people noticed the difference. When I eventually succumbed to one of the pretty acrylic wigs it looked terrific and I took a holiday to cover the change-over.

'It took courage to wear the new wig back at work but I felt so good in it, so modern and proud of myself, that I took the plunge. Two people have remarked that they like the new hair-style, so I think I've got away with it.

'There are a couple of people in the parish I would really like to tell about my hair, but the opportunity has not presented itself. Lying, covering up, makes you feel faintly guilty. I wonder all the time whether they suspect.'

Lesley feels she is missing out on a home and family, 'and wigs are not a great help. When I first went out with a chap I felt I had to explain about the wig before it was too late and he had knocked it off. He was a teacher — we got on well — but when he started to kiss me I had to stop him and explain.'

His reaction surprised her. 'The awful thing was that he thought it was a great joke. You'd have thought I was wearing a wig for fun. It was quite incredible the way he fell about laughing. He made joke after joke . . . and I had to listen to his endless cracks.

'He was buying a new house. There had been some serious talk about my living in it with him. But when we broke up he bought a picture of a woman with her wig rolling off. He said it reminded him of me.

'It shattered my confidence for further relationships. Many people can't cope with baldness. You must act out this pretence of having a head of hair to protect others.'

SHARON, who's a social worker, disagrees. At 30, she has now been telling people the truth for some years.

'When I first lost my hair severely, at 15, I lay on my bed and cried for hours. Every morning I would leap up and shove my wig on quickly so that I couldn't catch sight of myself in the mirror!

'I dreaded wearing it at school for the first time, but no one was cruel or poked fun at me. Maybe I was just lucky. Two specialists predicted my hair would be back "by the time I was 21". Not a bit of it, I'm afraid, and since the age of 22 I have had to wear a wig all the time.

'It's the "no one need know" argument that has been a problem for me. The less people know you wear a wig, the more alopecia becomes a guilty secret. You start to think "X likes me but he wouldn't if he knew I was bald."

'I realized recently that it was because so few people knew that I had begun to view my baldness as something to be ashamed of. So I started leaving my wig off more around the house. I started to mention to one or two colleagues at work that I wore a wig. They were interested, sympathetic, but certainly not shocked or horrified. One of them came up to me a couple of days ago and remarked "You know, you are lucky! I had to get up at six this morning to wash and set my hair!"'

Her breakthrough, she says, came the day she decided to show a man friend — 'I'm very fond of him' — what she looked like without a wig. 'Again, no shock or horror, just interest and concern, and he seems to have survived the ordeal. I'm not advocating that people should whip off their wigs at every possible moment saying "Look, everyone, I'm bald!" But if you choose your moment and your confidants, being open about it helps enormously. I've recently started self-defence classes and have had to mention I wear a wig in case it slips during a mock stranglehold!

'Being a social worker, I realize that some of the reason I didn't want people to know I was bald was that I like people to think of me as someone who copes with life, who is strong and not the least vulnerable. By saying to people, 'Well, actually, I'm bald,' what you're really saying is "Look, I'm vulnerable, just like you!"'

SARAH: *'I'm a hysteric. That's what they all think. She's lost all her hair — sign of hysteria!'*

Sarah, the sophisticate, had been used to having fun, plenty of men friends. As a nursing sister, she enjoyed the social life of the hospital. But, she says, losing her hair put paid to all that.

Her last steady man friend was a doctor, aged 42. 'He was kind, sensible, normal. We saw each other regularly for nine months. Everything was wonderful. There was just one thing he kept moaning about. He wanted me to take off my wig. I couldn't. I told him that I looked awful without it but he kept on.'

Sarah is 48 but looks much younger in her fashionable fair wigs. Her clothes are smart. She loves her country cottage, with its Laura Ashley prints and adoring Labradors.

She had been truthful with her man friend about her alopecia right from the start. At first, it didn't seem to matter. Sarah is the kind of attractive, trendy woman who can converse on nearly everything, bring joy and jokes to every situation. Any man would be proud to take her for a drink.

As their relationship became serious, she decided to comply with his request. 'In the end I thought, well it's silly to try to hide under a wig. If you're going to share a bed with someone, he will have to know sometime. So, one night, reluctantly, I took it off.

'It was the worst mistake I could have made. His face changed instantly. He looked disgusted. "My God", he said, "I had no idea you would look as revolting as that!" Then he sat down and remarked conversationally, "It really is repulsive, isn't it?"'

That was the end of the relationship. 'I finished with him after that.'

As a nurse, Sarah remembers trying to comfort mastectomy patients whose husbands couldn't help them. 'We would send a patient home after the trauma of losing a breast and her husband would refuse to look at her. He would switch off the light in the bedroom so he never had to see where she had been mutilated. It was always happening.

"Bastards", I used to think, "behaving like that to your poor wives." But I would say to the patient "Look, your husband has a problem. He feels threatened and insecure. You've got to be strong for both of you and help him through."

'Now here I was with a man who apparently felt threatened by the fact that I'd lost my hair. That was it, all over.'

She turned to a girl friend for reassurance. 'But she looked at my wig-less scalp and agreed. "Yes. It does look revolting, doesn't it?"'

Sarah longs for the thick hair she had in her teens. 'It was long and auburn, just like the Duchess of York's. But I had bald patches all through my nursing career. You can imagine what fun it was trying to balance a nurse's cap on top of a wig!'

In her early thirties her hair suddenly became worse. 'All my hair fell out soon after a break-in at home. The burglar tried to pin me down on the bed and sexually assaulted me, but you can't prove anything like that so he got away with it. He had a gun and I was terrified.'

A week or so later her patchy alopecia areata deteriorated into total scalp hair loss. 'My doctor told me I was hysterical and nothing could be done for me.'

That was 12 years ago, but when Sarah was recently injured in a road accident, the subject was dragged up again. 'In the court case afterwards, when I was trying to get some kind of compensation, an orthopaedic surgeon gave evidence about my injuries. He said "This woman has alopecia universalis so is clearly of a hysterical personality." This evidence was later challenged by a consultant dermatologist who said: "There are conflicting data on whether a dermatologist would accept that stress can precipitate this condition in predisposed individuals. I know of no good studies where a hysterical personality was thought to be important in pathogenesis — the origin and development of this disease." He added: "I think the orthopaedic surgeon was stepping out of his speciality a little bit in his comments."'

Sarah shares her home with a woman friend but still finds it difficult to meet strangers. 'People look at you and their eyeline rises to your "hair"! They know it is a wig and you feel inexplicably ashamed. I can be talking to someone normally and suddenly I notice that they are not talking to my eyes any longer but addressing their remarks to the crown of my head.

'I went out for a meal with some friends and the waiter was very chatty. He confided that he had once taken great pleasure in catching his cuff link deliberately in a customer's hair to dislodge her wig. He said, "I can tell a wig a mile off." Then, in front of every one, he turned to me and said "I knew hers was a wig and I know yours is too."'

Sarah feels that she has missed out on the chance of a husband and family.

'People think it's contagious. I hate having to explain because they make you feel you have something dirty and catching.

'I've never had any medical treatment for my hair. Just "Go home. Don't think about it. Wear a wig." On the rare occasions when I've been to bed with a man, I've always been terrified it would come off.

'I decided recently to have another attempt to make contacts and joined a computer dating agency. I had some phone calls from a very nice-sounding chap, a widower. We arranged to meet, but I did make a point of telling him I wore a wig beforehand.

'He didn't seem worried about it so I bought a new coat and got all dressed up to meet him. Then, just as I was leaving the house, the phone rang. He couldn't make it. I never heard from him again.'

Sarah has now resigned herself to a life without men. She enjoys the affection of a close woman friend and her dogs, 'but I wouldn't risk going out with another man. I've been hurt too much.'

MARIANNE: 'I am a fat freak. I was tossed on the scrap heap at a very early age.'

At 40, Marianne is still fat from the side-effects of the systemic steroids prescribed for her at 15. A teacher in Scotland, she has suffered from alopecia areata since she was 11.

'By the time I was 15 I had lost nearly all my hair. I took steroids for three years, put on 3 stones in weight, and ended up with a very round face, stretch marks all over my body, and serious kidney problems which landed me in hospital. The doctors immediately stopped the steroids and my hair started to fall out again. During the treatment it had been regrowing quite well. The doctors told me that my hair would never regrow. They were wrong. It has returned but nine times it has come out again.'

Marianne is bitter. She feels that the loss of her hair has contributed largely towards the isolation of the life she leads now, at home with her widowed mother, teaching locally.

'In the years following the systemic steroids, I tried various things: steroid injections into the scalp, and, most recently, minoxidil. I have had very little help from doctors and no sympathy whatsoever.

'I really feel very angry, not because I have an affliction — many people have handicaps — but because I feel that I was tossed on the scrap heap at a very early age. So much seems to be done for other people and nothing for me.

'I have always felt very bitter about people's reactions to me — I was called a fat freak! Nobody has ever tried to help me come to terms with a rather restricted life. I have never lost the weight I put on in my teens although I have tried many times. Being fat and bald has ruined my life. I'll never forget the people who made remarks at my expense, from my childhood onwards. Some of them were far from good-looking themselves. I don't have buck teeth or acne and I am of normal height.

'As a child, I remember grown-ups recoiling in horror. "Oh, but you were such a pretty little girl!" they used to say.'

By the time she started college at 18 she had to wear a wig. 'It made me shy, wearing a wig. All the students were having a great time except me. Saturday was always a bad time. I lived at home though others were sharing flats. I couldn't — everyone would have found out that I was bald.

'At college a girl pulled it off by mistake. She was so shocked they had to take her to hospital. Nobody asked how I felt.

'I've never had a very happy home life as my father was often ill. When I got alopecia I started to postpone everything in life "until my hair grows back". But it didn't — at least not for long — and here I am at 40 and I've lost the chance of marriage and children.

'Somehow I've never been able to enjoy myself. Going on holiday, for instance — what if I had to share a room? I could never relax and have a drink. If I got drunk, the wig might slip off. People would know.

'I don't get as emotional as I once did. After all, there is nobody to listen. But I do regret my lost youth.'

MERYL, at 39, also feels that alopecia has had a disastrous effect on her love life. She is a lecturer in biology and her career has always taken up a great deal of her time and concentration.

'My first bout of alopecia was at the age of 13 and just meant that my early experiences of boyfriends were delayed a few years. I was short, fat, wore glasses and was more interested in O levels anyway, so it didn't matter.

'Two further episodes in my twenties didn't worry me much either, as I was just starting a new job. Sex has never figured highly in my life. I am a friendly, cuddly person rather than passionate.'

But problems really began when her hair fell out again, in her thirties. 'I had met a man and started a relationship which was to last five years. He is in computers and travels around a lot. We spent every weekend together but kept our separate houses as our work was far apart.

'As my hair was gradually falling out I took to wearing scarves all the time, which I hated. But he never seemed to mind. I'd lost up to 60 per cent of my hair but the condition seemed to be improving so I started to leave off the scarves.

'I was trying on clothes in a changing room with mirrors all around. Suddenly I caught sight of the rear view and was horrified. I flipped through the yellow pages and found a new firm and my first wonderful wig. Is it like first love? I have such fond memories of that first one — so thick, curly and superb that it changed my attitudes and confidence overnight.'

But her lover's reaction was less than expected. 'What on earth is that?' he asked. 'I think it's dreadful.'

From then on our relationship went downhill. He refused to talk to me about it. Lovemaking turned into just having sex, until I felt I was just being used. Eventually I could take no more and we split up. I can only conclude that he was undermined by my new image and confidence. Did he want me more under control and so unattractive that no one else would want me? I felt like an Orthodox Jewish woman whose religious faith obliges her to wear a wig when she marries.

'Since then, I've been through terrible depressions about never having a loving sexual relationship again. At 39, I cannot think how I would bring up the subject to someone I cared about. I feel vulnerable, even ugly.

'I have several men friends who keep suggesting taking me to bed — men always feel obliged to try at least — and, much as I might be tempted, I hold back and keep them at arm's length.

'I realize that this is not an awful illness. It is all psychological and other people are in a lot worse situations. But until I can come to terms with things I shall continue to envy couples and come home from parties alone.'

Perhaps because of the repeated disappointments of this eccentric disease, many people lose heart. Their hair falls out, grows back, and then, as often as not, falls out again. It's hard to take psychologically, but some have found that the right approach makes all the difference.

SUSANNAH, *young West End secretary, enjoyed her Saturday nights in the cheerful company of her colleagues and flatmates.*

It had been a good party. The young man who had taken her home was warm and affectionate. 'Very dishy indeed,' she thought, as his hands ran admiringly over her slim figure. A trendy girl, at 24, her light brown hair was mousse-moulded into fashionable spikes.

The handsome young graduate leaned towards her on the sofa, his fingers eager on the buttons of her dress . . . Susannah pulled away sharply, shattering his mood.

'What's the matter?' He was disappointed, wondering what he had done. Susannah felt downcast, her joy evaporating. She had remembered just in time, before he found out for himself. Her hair, her bloody, bloody hair . . .

Susannah lost her hair at 23. In three months, small bald patches developed into total loss. The first thing it wrecked was her sex life.

'At first, I didn't tell people. Unless there was some reason for them to know I didn't see why I should tell them. With men, I tried to tell them before things got close and there was imminent danger that they would knock the wig off my head. The first chap I told — it was awful. It took me ages to tell him. I was afraid he would jump back in horror, make an excuse and leave . . . or whatever men do in these circumstances.' She hesitated so long that she was finally obliged to tell him in the middle of a passionate embrace. 'He laughed, actually. He was amazed that I had made so much fuss about it. We went on to have quite a good relationship which, in the end, I finished myself.'

When she lost her hair, she had thought it was the end of any normal sex life. 'I was wrong. I have had three serious men friends since then and I'm now happily married. Other women ought to know that losing your hair is not the end of any chance of being happy.'

She saw an endocrinologist very early in her treatment. 'He said, "It is unlikely your hair will ever grow back." At that stage I had been losing it over a few months and I hadn't made a fuss, but when he said that, I cried. I couldn't face going back to my office that afternoon. I went home and sobbed for three days. In the end my mother, very worried about me, came to my room and said "Look, you are going to be all right. You can still have an attractive appearance. You are just going to work harder at it." '

By the end of that week, Susannah stopped crying and made a few decisions. Being a strong-minded girl, she decided that she enjoyed her job, working in the office of a whisky company. She loved the social life of the West End, and she would try to ensure that her baldness made as little difference as possible.

'I continued going to parties. I bought a selection of brightly coloured berets and arranged the hair I had left around the edges of them. I didn't go to parties specifically to meet men, just to enjoy myself. As it happened, I did meet men and make new relationships. I was surprised. My lack of hair didn't put them off.'

She also found a range of wigs which she really liked. 'They were very expensive. I spent £1,400 but they were worth it. When they were discontinued in the UK I had to send to Germany for them.'

After she had told the first man about her hair loss, the relationship continued, 'but we were not really well suited. I was terrified he would leave me because I didn't think anyone else would want me. So I was clinging to him. He said it didn't matter. But the more my hair fell out, the more depressed I became and I think it did affect him a bit. I wasn't my usual cheerful self.

'In the end my mother saw what was happening and pointed out that I was clutching at straws. I decided to end the relationship and felt much better when he had gone — though I did think "That's it. I've throw away my last chance."'

Eventually, she met up with the man who became her husband. He had known her several years earlier, before she lost her hair. He was complimentary, boosting her morale by saying he actually preferred the short wig. 'I let him see me without a wig straight away. I wanted to say "This is me, like it or lump it!" When we first got together my hair was starting to grow back, but it has all fallen out again so I am back to square one. At home I wear turbans in the evenings and in bed.

'Now we're married I won't let him see my scalp. I'm more embarrassed about it than I was before. I suppose I'm less optimistic than I was at first. This disease seems to recur so often you begin to lose heart.

'But a woman need never be afraid that no man will want her. You have to decide not to let this ruin your life. You must not let it stop you doing things. You have to be positive. I was married six months ago – in a wig – and we are very happy.'

Survival plan

You are single. Your hair – or most of it – has gone, so has your confidence. Male or female, there are two ingredients you need in your life now.

The first is a friend, someone close to you, willing to listen endlessly to your worries without getting bored – or at least not showing it! Someone who can reassure, lie and lie and lie and say that your hair *will* return. At the beginning you need to believe that your hair is coming back. Later you may become accustomed to the thought that it might not, but not at the beginning.

There are friends and friends. You don't want the competitive kind who will see this as the opportunity to be one up on you at last, who looks at you, losing your hair at 33, and says blithely, 'Well, of course, it is all caused by the menopause.' You do not need that kind of friend. But everyone needs a confiding relationship.

The second necessity is a good wig, for a woman, anyway. A man may prefer to sport the Kojak look. For a woman, a wig is a top priority. There may be days when you rebel and want to walk around with a naked head. Fine, but for everyday life, you're going to be forced to conform to some extent. For a 'normal' job or 'normal' social life, a wig is essential.

Then the worrying begins. The first thought in a new relationship is: 'How do I break the news that I'm wearing a wig?' The second little niggle which sabotages peace of mind is: 'Can he/she tell it's a wig, anyway?' You fret. You let it ruin the anticipatory excitement of the first weeks of any new relationship. You are too concerned about choosing the right moment, preferably before the wretched thing is knocked off and it is too late for subterfuge.

Stop it. Remember Susannah who said: 'When I finally broke it to him, after weeks of anxiety, he just laughed and said "Is that all?"'

You may, of course, be unlucky and get one of the types who can't take it. If he is so insecure that he feels threatened by baldness in a woman, do you really want him anyway? The men who are big enough to cope with it are the *only* ones worth having, not that such a thought will be much comfort to you at the time. It may be years before you realize just what a wimp he was.

Being unmarried, you need never fear that your boyfriend or girlfriend stayed with you because he or she was married to you already, and had no choice.

Being without hair will only ruin your life if you let it, if you make it the obstacle which prevents you doing things, if you become Miss Negative – you know the sort. Every time anyone makes a suggestion you give it an instant veto. 'No, I couldn't do that . . . because of my hair.'

Be positive. College lecturer Susan Crabtree from Burnley, Lancashire, who lost all her hair when her children were small, found it helped a lot to realize how much better her wigs looked than most people's hair-styles. 'It helped me most to find a really beautiful wig in just the right shade. I know now that my "hair" will always look good, when I want it to, whatever happens. It boosts me most when strangers ask where I have my hair done!'

She has been asked to take over the hairdressing class at her technical college. 'I was even asked by the principal whether I would let the students practise hairdressing on my own hair! I laughed. "Yes", I said, "if they can find it!"'

But I can't wear a wig *all* the time, you groan. Of course you can't, but don't forget that bald can be beautiful. A young woman I know lost all her hair in the space of two months. She came to a Hairline meeting at my house where we were all decorously clad in our wigs. But the spring afternoon grew warm. Soon she had had enough and tossed the wig across the room. 'It's so sticky. Let's relax,' she said.

We were all amazed. Her hairless head was revealed as one of the most beautifully shaped I have ever seen, pretty, vulnerable, far from repulsive. Her husband, who married her in the days when she had hair, still thinks she is the most attractive girl in the world.

Marilyn, a young Bristol mum who lost her hair, says: 'We used to go around in a foursome with another couple. Now I'm bald, the other chap makes it a bit embarrassing because he once saw me without my wig and says he fancies me. When I had hair he never gave me a second glance!'

A Parisian model shaved her head one year for the winter collections. She was the toast of Paris. No one was photo-

graphed more. Years later, when I was among the press corps
covering the shows we were all hoping some model would
do the same. It was a sensational story and she was a sensational girl. Sex appeal? Fantastic, agreed the photographers,
and they are a fussy breed.

More recently, singer Sinead O'Connor shaved her head
and looked so attractive that a few of her fans were moved to
do the same.

The fashionable in Britain began buying a new type of wig,
a hairless skin which fits tightly over a head of hair to make a
normal head appear bald, like the scalp skins used in films
and TV. Pieces of false hair could be attached to this in
switches to achieve a new look. Who knows? If this goes on,
other women may soon be copying *us* and shaving their heads
instead of going to the hairdresser. I'm joking, of course . . .
but fashions in beauty change and things could just swing our
way!

If you are young and trendy you may decide this is your
opportunity to buy a sensational wardrobe of wigs – purple,
pink, gold silver, yellow – and wear a different one for every
day of the week. If you can carry it off, why not?

Whatever you do, don't despair! Being hairless needn't
stop you marrying, as Susannah did, building a career, or
doing anything in life you really want to.

PART III

Treatments

7

WHAT TREATMENTS ARE AVAILABLE?

'There must be something we can do . . .
some kind of medical help.'

There are several medical treatments currently available for alopecia areata/totalis/universalis. No one pretends they are cures. The aim is to persuade the hair to grow – if not permanently, then at least as a stopgap until it regrows spontaneously.

Treatments include:

A For less severe cases, where hair loss is less than 60 per cent of all scalp hair:

- Minoxidil (in solution applied to the scalp); other vasodilators also used topically
- Steroid creams or lotions rubbed into the affected areas. An example is Betnovate
- Dithranol/Anthralin
- Injections into the scalp of steroid (intra-lesional corticosteroids)

B For more severe cases, where the hair loss is more than 60 per cent of all scalp hair:

- Counter-irritants or contact allergens applied to the affected area to induce an eczema-like response. Examples are dinitrochlorobenzene (DNCB), diphencyprone, and *Primula obconica* combined with systemic steroids by injection/ACTH (or corticotrophin, a hormone)
- Steroids by mouth
- PUVA
- Immuno-suppressive drugs, as used in transplant surgery, such as Cyclosporine, usually applied topically, in gel form, and Azathioprine, occasionally used orally in cases where other treatments have failed.

Minoxidil

'Mummy, you're turning into a teddy bear!' said my six-year-old daughter, tracing the tiny white hairs sprouting on my cheeks. Below the ears, there was also a sudden growth of vellous, downy hair, a shadow above my lips, too. A Zapata moustache, I thought, any minute now . . .

'Doctor', I murmured, 'I'm growing a beard'. The dermatologist smiled. 'Oh, well . . . it proves minoxidil works, doesn't it?'

Four years after I first lost my hair, when it was beginning to grow back, but agonizingly slowly, I hear the news that minoxidil, a drug used in the treatment of high blood pressure, had been found, by accident, to make hair grow as a side-effect. An elderly lady in Colorado was amazed when the tablets she had been prescribed for her blood pressure gave her the added bonus of a moustache. Young men who had been depressed about their hair loss were delighted when it grew back, all thanks to minoxidil, a vasodilator – a drug used to dilate the blood vessels – which they had been given to lower their blood pressure.

It was marketed under the name Loniten by its manufacturers, the Upjohn Company, from their giant pharmaceutical plant in Kalamazoo, Michigan. For several years, this highly respectable company ignored the drug's potential for growing hair. It was not keen on anything so cosmetic as a 'cure for baldness': its reputation hinged on serious medicine. But news of the hair-growth factor leaked when a cardiac physician, Dr Anthony Zappacosta, reported in the *New England Journal of Medicine* that one of his patients, a bald man of 38, had regrown hair while taking the drug for his heart condition.[21]

Dermatologists were soon involved in world-wide trials. They applied a solution containing a tiny percentage of minoxidil to the scalp. Volunteer guinea pigs – all with balding heads – queued up to try it in the USA, Denmark, the UK, all of them desperate to find out whether the miracle worked.

I was a guinea pig in the UK, prescribed minoxidil at one of London's teaching hospitals: first, a two per cent solution, then three per cent. Soon tiny hairs appeared in the bald patches on my scalp. They also grew a little on my face. The doctor thought I had splashed it too generously on my scalp and it had run down the sides of my face. The hair had grown there, just as it had on my face. He added that usually the drug only made hair grow in the wrong places when taken by mouth.

I was not complaining! I was delighted that the solution was helping to thicken up the regrowth on my scalp. In any case, the facial hair soon disappeared.

But what was the minoxidil miracle all about? Everyone was asking about it.

Some doctors hailed it as a breakthrough. The widespread research it prompted could only be a good thing and encourage more medical interest in alopecia areata. The minoxidil saga, said the doctors, is a modern fairy tale.

Minoxidil: a Modern Fairy Tale

Once upon a time, there were hundreds of women hiding away from the world, because they felt they were freaks. They had been normal. They had been pretty. Until suddenly, for no reason they knew of, they lost their hair.

Doctors couldn't help, knowing neither cause nor cure. 'Wear a wig', they told the Cinderellas. 'It's a shame about these unfortunate women', they told each other, 'but it doesn't hurt, won't kill them and we have more important sicknesses to cure'.

They couldn't help the bald men, either. The young princes should have been Prince Charmings but their scalps were patchy with alopecia. They were so disgusted with the way they looked that they had lost 'that loving feeling'! They looked in the mirror and thought that no Cinderella would ever go to the ball with them.

The Cinderellas went home and managed as best they could. They hid under wigs and scarves. They stayed in their kitchens and stopped wanting to go out. They were afraid their husbands wouldn't want them any more.

Some wore their wigs in bed. Some smacked their children when they knew they shouldn't. Some took to drink.

The balding Prince Charmings stayed home too, afraid their princesses would laugh at them as they had no hirsute manliness to offer. They were lonely.

Then along came the Fairy Godmother. She waved her magic wand and a quite ordinary little drug suddenly started to make hair grow again. It was called minoxidil. Doctors grew keen and fascinated. Men with money saw the opportunities in a cure for baldness. Massive injections of pharmaceutical cash were pumped into research.

The Cinderellas and the Prince Charmings were delighted because at last someone was taking an interest in their problem. Whether it worked or not, minoxidil could be the key to future research. 'In other words', said the Cinderellas, 'this is a breakthrough.'

Some of them even went to the ball . . .

It may sound like a fairy tale, but it has certainly triggered more interest in research into alopecia.

It attracts some important questions.

How Was Minoxidil's Potential for Hair Growth Discovered?

Over 25 years ago, minoxidil began life as a metabolite, a breakdown product extracted from rats' urine, intended as an anti-ulcer medication which would act on gastric solutions.

But it was more use to the heart than the stomach, discovered its manufacturers, the Upjohn Company, a pharmaceutical firm founded over a hundred years ago by Dr William Erasmus Upjohn, whose grandfather was English. They soon found out that it was a strong vasodilator, funded research, and by 1979 the USA Food and Drugs Administration (FDA) approved its use for the treatment of high blood pressure, under the trade name of Loniten.

But during these trials some patients grew hair in odd places. A young doctor experimented privately by making up a solution of crushed minoxidil tablets and applying it to the heads of his bald friends. He took out a patent on its use as a hair restorer.

The company apologized to the FDA for the incident and took out a separate hair use patent, promising that, in future, it would be used only as a blood pressure drug; but heart physician Dr Zappacosta's sudden revelation in the medical press dragged the subject into the open again.

Upjohn launched trials into minoxidil's use as a hair restorer. It was tested on macaque monkeys, who usually lose their hair at adolescence. Three out of four adult monkeys ended up with thickening hair. State prisoners volunteered to take part in the trials, as did thousands in hospitals in New York and Washington. Cosmetically significant regrowth was reported in about a third of volunteers.

How Is Minoxidil Used?

For clinical trials, hospitals made up their own preparations: a tiny percentage of the drug (from 1 to 5 per cent) in an alcohol solution. The patient applies this to the bald area twice daily.

How Soon Can Regrowth Be Expected?

Within four months . . . if it is going to work in your case! Dermatologist Dr John Wilkinson cautions: 'It is *not* a cure for baldness and it appears that only one in three patients obtains significant benefit. It is also expensive.'

Does Minoxidil Work for Everyone?

No. Clinical trials have found that it works best on early male pattern baldness and patchy alopecia areata. It has not been very successful on totally bald heads. In a major British trial, Dr David Fenton of St Thomas's Hospital, London, and Dr John Wilkinson of the Wycombe General Hospital, High Wycombe, concluded: 'Although we have little doubt that topical minoxidil can induce new hair growth in patients with alopecia areata, those with more severe and extensive disease have a worse response. Those with alopecia universalis and alopecia totalis may not respond at all.'[22]

Using a 1 per cent solution of minoxidil, this study found that, at six months, 81 per cent of patients were responding. After a year, 50 to 70 per cent of those with patchy alopecia areata had some regrowth; 60 per cent had 'cosmetically acceptable' hair growth – they had no need of a wig.

Other area results included:

• DENMARK[23]

One of the four cases of patchy alopecia grew 'cosmetically satisfying' hair. She could discard her wig. Twenty-three patients were involved but the other 19 had extended or total hair loss. Thirteen out of the 23 had some regrowth (1 per cent minoxidil).

• UNITED KINGDOM

Manchester[24] Two out of four patients with patchy alopecia areata had complete recovery. There was no success with cases of total hair loss (3 per cent minoxidil).

Liverpool[25] Out of nine patients, one grew sufficient hair to discard her wig (1 per cent minoxidil), but these were all patients with extensive or total hair loss where it was known that the outlook was not so hopeful (from the Fenton/Wilkinson trial).

Aberdeen[26] Nineteen out of 28 patients with patchy alopecia areata showed regrowth, including one 'striking case of unilateral terminal hair regrowth' (1 per cent minoxidil). Doctors' verdict: 'worthy of further evaluation.'

Sunderland[27] An 80 per cent success rate in regrowing the hair of 53 patients, including one with total loss.

- **USA**
  Chicago, 1981[28] Two cases of total hair loss had complete regrowth (1 per cent minoxidil). The regrowth occurred in a girl of 13 and a woman of 42.
  Chicago, 1984[29] Twenty-five out of 48 patients had regrowth. Of those, 11 had 'cosmetically acceptable' hair. Two patients from this group who had total hair loss regrew it successfully (1 per cent minoxidil). Later research here reported achieving a better quality of hair with 5 per cent minoxidil. [30]
- In the treatment of androgenic – male pattern – baldness, the Upjohn Company reported a success rate of 76 per cent after more than 2,000 patients had been closely monitored for a year.

Is Minoxidil Safe?

For a 1 per cent topical solution, Fenton/Wilkinson, UK, said: 'so far no side-effects'. Dr John Wilkinson adds: 'Long-term risks have yet to be established'. Chicago reported 'no side-effects', and Sunderland's verdict was 'safe, convenient and effective'.

Mild skin irritations were reported in one study in America. Two Aberdeen patients had to give up the treatment due to dermatitis. Doctors wondered whether the fact that they were wearing wigs was connected.

A Manchester woman on 3 per cent minoxidil developed palpitations and chest pain but recovered when returned to 1 per cent.[31] Doctors suggested she might have been applying the lotion too liberally with the customary enthusiasm of alopecia patients. They advised caution in the use of higher concentrations of minoxidil in patients with extensive alopecia areata and those with known coronary heart disease.

No patients died during the trials but five deaths were

reported in America among the thousand who continued using it under their own doctor's supervision.

There were also five further deaths, two in Upjohn alopecia areata studies and two among users of non-Upjohn minoxidil formulations. The tenth death was that of a man who had been in a study for patients taking blood pressure drugs by mouth. He was on active drugs for 16 days then dropped out of the study. He died two months later.

It was quite clear that all the deaths were caused by reasons other than the patients' use of minoxidil, the causes including such serious conditions as AIDS and heart — cardio-vascular — complaints. The patients' use of minoxidil was purely coincidental and any public scares about the drug were quite unjustified!

All the cases were reported to the American Food and Drug Administration and Upjohn says that minoxidil did *not* have anything to do with the deaths.

The volunteers underwent exhaustive medical checks throughout the trials. While patients on the 3 per cent concentration had higher minoxidil blood levels than those on the 2 per cent, observed levels were low and not clini-cally significant.

Once I Start Using Minoxidil, Do I Have to Go on Using It Forever?

In some cases, yes. Some men who have male pattern bald-ness find they need to continue using it after their hair has regrown. Some have found that their hair drops out again when they stop, usually four months afterwards. In patients with alopecia areata, it is hoped that minoxidil will act as a stopgap measure to see them through until spontaneous regrowth occurs — so that they can stop using it.

How Does Minoxidil Work?
Several possibilities have been suggested:

- Minoxidil has a suppressive effect on the overworking immune system and thereby puts an end to the overkill mechanism which is operating on the hair follicles. In some research, minoxidil appeared to act on the lymphocyte accumulation surrounding the hair follicle.
- Minoxidil also seems to affect the size of hair follicles so that they return to their normal diameter and depth. Hair follicles in alopecia areata are usually much reduced in size.
- As the drug is a vasodilator, it has been suggested that it dilates the blood vessels around the hair follicles and stimulates growth.
- It may stimulate the hair to go into a growth – anagen – phase of its cycle, instead of a telogen – resting – phase.

How Can I Get Minoxidil?
The Upjohn Company has a minoxidil solution on the market, under the name of Regaine (Rogaine in Canada). It has 2 per cent concentration.

Why Has Minoxidil Been So Difficult to Get?
The system of registration for drugs in most countries demands that a company demonstrate the safety and efficacy of the product for a specific indication. Although minoxidil was already in use world-wide as a drug for high blood pressure, a separate set of clinical trials had to be completed for its use in hair growth. This took a long time, then the medical authorities in each country had to consider it, so for two or three years it had to play the waiting game in countries such as Britain and America. Belgium and Canada were among the first to give it the OK.

During this time, it was possible to get minoxidil through the health service in the UK on an individual patient/consultant basis, but often only where the hospital was involved in trials.

Should I Buy It through One of the Non-medical 'Clinics' – the Commercial Set-ups – Who Advertise It?

Only if you are a millionaire! As Upjohn's patent ran out in October 1986, and the company was still awaiting the DSS go-ahead from the Committee on the Safety of Medicines, many commercial enterprises saw their opportunity and bought the drug from abroad to sell privately – at at price! At one commercial 'clinic' I was offered a three-month supply of the drug for £395 and was informed by the counsellor that I would never get it from my own doctor. This is not true.

The DSS expressed concern at the increase in these clinics and suggested that they could be in breach of the Medicines Act. This lays down that a product can only be used for the purpose for which it was granted.

Why is Minoxidil Officially Prescribed for Male Pattern/Common Baldness and Not Alopecia Areata?

Because the trials for its use in common/male pattern baldness were completed when the company applied for its registration. Trials to test its use in alopecia areata and female pattern baldness were still in progress.

Meanwhile, a British doctor could prescribe it for someone with AA if he or she thought it would benefit the patient, but as this did not follow the officially approved indications, the responsibility for its use rested with the doctor and not the company. If anything went wrong, it would be on his or her own head!

Topical minoxidil (Regaine) became licensed for prescription for hair loss in 1988 (for men), 1990 (for women). It was available only on private prescription in the UK, at a cost of around £30 until 1995.

Does Minoxidil (Regaine) Work?

Many patients with thinning hair or less severe alopecia areata have found that Regaine helps. Some dermatologists favour a higher percentage solution of the drug – up to 5 per cent. Some also use it with retinoic acid (vitamin A).

KARLA lives in Belgium. Her hair started falling out after the birth of her seond child and she lost at least half of it, as diffuse alopecia, leaving it sparse and thin.

As soon as Regaine was licensed in Belgium, she started a course and after four months saw considerable improvement, 'not exactly regrowth but somehow the existing hair had become thicker and the parting much less obvious. Fewer hairs were being shed.

'After seven month, I decided to stop Regaine as I reckoned there had been sufficient improvement. Alas, three to four months later the fall-out began again and my hair is thinning drastically.

'They did warn me in the Regaine leaflet that this might happen and I am now wondering whether to return to it. It is expensive – the equivalent of about £30 for a month's supply in Belgium – but I am lucky enough to have it reimbursed under my medical insurance scheme. It looks as though I will have to go on using it for a very long time'.

ALEX, a London secretary, had lost all her hair but had been lucky enough to have complete regrowth. When she noticed a small bald patch she was horrified, thinking that she was going to lose all her hair again. She was prescribed minoxidil and found that it did seem to help the small patch clear up again.

But it did not work for Anna, who had lost all her hair, nor for Rowena, who had also lost all scalp hair.

ROWENA was so desperate to get her hair back that she was prepared to try almost anything. She was in her early twenties and engaged to a young doctor 'but I was putting off everything, including marriage, until there was some hope of getting my hair back'.

A course of steroid tablets had left her 3 stones overweight. In desperation she went to one of the commercial 'clinics', where she was offered minoxidil in a cream form. It cost her £395, 'but I didn't have any sign of hair. Not one! The doctor I saw at the clinic wasn't too interested in talking about minoxidil. He was too busy telling me to go on a diet. I began to wonder if he was being paid commission by the manufacturers of the diet he kept recommending!'

Having been available only on private prescription in the UK since 1988, in January 1995 Regaine (topical minoxidil) received the go-ahead to be sold over the pharmacist's counter. This is a ruling by the UK Committee on the Safety of Medicines who include it in a batch of prescription-only medicines released to be sold over the UK counter. The committee recommended only that Regaine (ie the two per cent minoxidil solution) be available in this way.

If patients want a treatment with a stronger solution of minoxidil (ie three, four or five per cent) this would have to be prescribed by a doctor.

Other vasodilators
On an experimental basis, other vasodilators, such as Viprostol, are also being tried.

Steroid creams or ointments

Other treatments for less severe alopecia areata include a steroid cream (such as Betnovate) rubbed into the bald patches: the patient rubs it into the scalp nightly.

Dithranol/Anthralin

This has been used with some success. A tar-like cream, often used to treat psoriasis, it is rubbed into the skin and left for a few hours before being washed off.

Injections of cortisone into the scalp (corticosteroids)

The injections are usually done about once a month, into the bald patches. This method works best when there is just a small area of baldness, or when the injections are done to encourage eyebrows to regrow.

For severe cases, where hair loss is more than 60 per cent, the following treatments are used:

Primary irritants

It all began with an onion . . . for years all kinds of unlikely substances were rubbed on the scalp in the hope of upsetting the skin, to make it so red and angry that the hair would be stimulated into growth. The ideal was a painful 'burn' on the skin. Sometimes the onion (or whatever) was rubbed in with a stiff brush! By the end of the 1960s doctors lost interest in these irritants. Their treatment wasn't doing any harm but it wasn't doing much good either.

On the other hand, allergen contact sensitizers are back in fashion again, now more is known about the immunology of alopecia areata. The idea is to use a substance to which the patient has become allergic.

The hope is that the lymphocytes – the white blood cells of the immune system – will switch to attacking this substance instead of the hair follicles, so that the hair is left to grow normally.

Consultant dermatologist Dr J. A. Savin of Edinburgh, writing in the *British Medical Journal* in 1982, asked whether the wheel had turned full circle with the return of these uncomfortable treatments.[32] 'Lymphocytes make up the bulk of the spectacular infiltrate to be seen in the early stages of this condition', he said, 'hanging like swarms of bees around the hair bulb'.

At that time, West German researchers were using the strong contact sensitizer dinitrochlorobenzene (DNCB) in this way. They were hoping, said Dr Savin, to stimulate lymphocyte accumulation in the scalp and so eliminate the stimulus producing their aggregation. DNCB was also used in the UK but there were worries about its possible mutagenicity. This led to the use of other powerful allergens. One of the most hopeful was diphencyprone/diphenylocyclopropenone.

Diphencyprone/diphenylcyclopropenone

Diphencyprone is an organic phenol derivative first used by West German dermatologist Dr Rudolph Happie. The solution is painted on to the heads of patients every week in the hope of producing an allergic reaction.

Dermatologist Dr Barry Monk, formerly of King's College Hospital, London, now at Bedford, presented a paper to the Royal Society of Medicine about his work with diphencyprone. Out of thirteen patients, five had successful hair regrowth, though it was rather patchy. Some of the successful cases had lost all their hair.

Many doctors see diphencyprone as a hopeful treatment because it is a harmless, non-toxic sensitizer. At Leeds General Infirmary it has been used on 29 patients of all ages, including a boy of 10, and induced hair growth in a woman who had had alopecia totalis for 54 years. 'Regrowth after such a long time really improves the patients' morale', says dermatologist Dr Susan Macdonald Hull, who worked on the trials. 'Fifty per cent of the patients showed some regrowth and 29 per cent had a cosmetically acceptable regrowth and could discard their wigs.'

LINDA rang me in tears when she first lost her hair. 'I have hardly any hair at all now and it took me four visits to my doctor to get an appointment with a dermatologist. Now, after waiting weeks to see him all the specialist can say is that nothing can be done.'

Shortly afterwards, however, her dermatologist offered her the chance to be a guinea pig in experimental work on diphencyprone at his hospital. 'The doctors explained that the idea is to get the body's immune system to attack the drug instead of the hair follicles, i.e. induce the body to become allergic to it.'

Linda is 33 and had lost her hair rapidly in less than a year. After two months' treatment, there was no success apart from a mild itching for about 48 hours afterwards. After four months, hair began to grow on the treated side of her head, 'but within two weeks it had all vanished. We persevered and after four months regrowth began and never stopped. Now both sides of my head are being treated and are beginning to even up. My hair is growing back the same dark brown colour it was before. I'll soon be able to go without a wig!'

JEAN has also been receiving diphencyprone treatment. She is 49 and has suffered from alopecia areata since she was 16, finally losing all her hair after she left a job in a printing firm, when the heavy lifting became too much for her.

When diphencyprone was first painted on to her head she says: 'My scalp felt rather sore for a few days and I had a feeling of swollen glands. This made me ill at first but the doctors made up a very weak solution. Then they strengthen it each week if it has not been too itchy.'

After four months' treatment, Jean has a short growth of hair on the side of her head which has been treated. The other (untreated) side is still bald.

'Last week, for the first time, they treated all my head so we shall wait and hope something happens! I'm keeping my fingers and toes crossed!'

Jean is convinced that worry about leaving her printing job aggravated her alopecia. She now has a part-time job in a residential home for the handicapped and is much happier.

Primula obconica

DORIS, 40, a school dinner lady, was very upset when she lost all her hair. She was a little surprised too, in a hospital skin clinic when the consultant dermatologist instructed her to strap a leaf of the Primula obconica to her arm! The leaf was changed every few days and replaced with a new one. Soon the skin on her arm became red and angry. The leaf was removed from her arm and rubbed on her head. After a month, Doris was amazed to see that hair was growing again!

The leaf treatment was combined with injections of ACTH (corticotrophin, the hormone of the anterior pituitary gland). It specifically stimulates the adrenal cortex to produce cortisol. These injections have to be carefully monitored as side-effects include weight gain.

Doris put on 2 stones in weight but her hair was marvellous. She had no need of a wig for eight years. She then had a relapse and was losing her hair again. This time her doctor used diphencyprone as a sensitizer and the hair is regrowing once more.

'I have never known it to grow so fast,' says Doris. 'In a month or so I'll be able to go around without a wig. My husband thinks it's smashing. I feel much better — the children at school don't call me "baldie" now!'

It may sound like modern witchcraft or something out of the Dark Ages but the amazing thing is that this leaf treatment actually seems to work, at least for some.

Dr E. L. Rhodes is a consultant dermatologist in Surrey. She pioneered work with the primula plant and published her research in the *British Journal of Dermatology*.[33] Dr Rhodes says that she came upon the idea while thinking of ways to induce an allergic response. 'I knew that some people are terribly allergic to *Primula obconica* and it seemed the answer'.

She has been pleased with the results. 'In my experience about a third of patients can regain their hair with primula sensitization and weekly injections of ACTH. The plant must be *Primula obconica* – only available from a florist. The common plant primula won't do it !'

Steroids by mouth

Sometimes patients with extensive loss of scalp hair are prescribed systemic steroids (taken by mouth), but these need to be carefully monitored by the dermatologist as possible side-effects include increased appetite and weight gain, plus, in long-term use, a greater susceptibility to high blood pressure, diabetes and brittle bone conditions.

Says consultant dermatologist Dr David Fenton: 'I like to discuss with the patient the various treatment options available so that together we can decide which is most suitable. Systemic steroids in short bursts can control active alopecia – an episode of alopecia when it is really raging.' He has also achieved regrowth using combination treatment – such as systemic steroids, such as prednisolone, Regaine (topical minoxidil) and zinc. This treatment has been successful even in cases of total hair loss.

KATY is in her early twenties and had lost all her body hair. It is regrowing well after four months and she has so far had no side-effects. She is still on the steroids.

PUVA therapy

PUVA treatment is time-consuming, as it involves two to five sessions a week, and no results can be expected before at least 20 sesssions. It is a pleasant treatment, popular with patients, as it involves exposure to long-wave ultraviolet light.

The patient has to take a sensitizing drug – psoralens – before the sessions and, as skin is sensitive to sunshine for a day or so afterwards, must be careful to keep out of direct sunlight for a short time.

Dr Sylvia Marston runs a Harley Street PUVA clinic. She says: 'It is very much a second-line treatment, mainly for some-one who has plenty of time to spare and is happy with just temporary regrowth. It is common for the regrown hair to dis-appear when treatment stops. There is also controversy about possible side-effects, such as skin problems and eye trouble'.

ROXANNE went to a private clinic for her PUVA treatment as her husband was in a medical insurance scheme. She says: 'I thoroughly enjoyed the treatment and hair was coming back nicely all over my head – where I had lost most of it. But during the course of treat-ments I discovered I was pregnant and had to give it up. I was rather concerned that the sensitizing drug might have affected the baby.'

The baby was fine; Roxanne's hair was not. It fell out again a few months after she gave birth.

PUVA is available under the NHS at some UK hospitals, though it is primarily used for psoriasis patients.

Immuno-suppressive drugs

Doctors know how to suppress the immune system to prevent it from rejecting transplanted organs, such as hearts and kidneys, after transplant surgery. So could immuno-suppressive drugs be used to prevent the immune system from rejecting the hair as foreign?

In theory, *yes*, says Dr David Fenton. In practice he is doubtful about the advisability of any interference with the immune system which might occur if the drugs were taken orally. 'They could cause the patient to become very ill,' he says. 'He or she might have severely lowered resistance to infection, possibly even a susceptibility to tumours.'

He has used the immuno-supprevise drug azathioprine orally only occasionally in cases where other treatments have failed, and only when very carefully monitored for side-effects.

Another immuno-suppressive drug, cyclosporine, has been the subject of research at a Surrey hospital to find out whether it will help hair regrow when applied *topically*, i.e. to the scalp in a 10 per cent gel. Dermatologist Dr Ian Coulsen has said 'We were impressed with results in France where it worked for eight out of nine patients. Used like this, the risks are minimized and so far there have been no side-effects on kidneys or blood pressure, though our research is still at an early stage.' It has been known for some years that cyclosporine promotes hair growth as a side-effect with transplant patients. Although the most recent trials have been disappointing, a hair grown in a test-tube by scientists at Cambridge University responded well to cyclosporine.

Current research is investigating the hair growth potential of Finasteride, a drug used in the treatment of male prostate problems and found to promote hair growth as a side-effect.

The thymus gland is known to be involved in hair growth. Some alopecia patients have been found to have a decreased level of thymulin in their bloodstream, and some workers are carrying out research into the link between low thymulin levels and hair loss.

8

WHAT ABOUT SURGERY?

*'But I'm really desperate.
What about surgery?'*

When people are desperate – as alopecia victims often are – the field is wide open for commercial firms to cash in. But no matter how depressed you are by the lack of medical help available, beware the high-street salon which offers a 'miracle' answer. *There are no miracle cures.*

Transplant surgery has been around for many years and has helped many men who needed to look presentable for the sake of their jobs – salesmen, actors, TV presenters – but the cost is high and the operation *must* be performed by a reputable doctor. Please don't get involved with the Sunday paper ads and the discreetly lit upmarket city salon. You need the advice of your own doctor and a dermatologist. With any luck he or she will be able to assess whether your baldness is seriously affecting you – whether you are depressed by it, whether it has become a serious handicap in your life.

It is, of course, usually the *man* with common or male pattern baldness who can be helped by a surgical transplant. In men or women with alopecia areata or general thinning this type of surgery is not normally feasible as the thinning is not confined to one area.

This surgery is controversial, anyway. Mr John Firmage of the Institute of Trichologists says: 'The effect on the scalp of many of these procedures can be horrific. I have seen scarring and infections. Be very, very careful'.

There are several kinds of treatment, including:

- Micro-grafting. This is the newest breakthrough in hair transplanting. Micro-plants, i.e. single hairs, are individually planted into slight nicks in the skin – one hair at a time. This gives a much more natural appearance than the older techniques, which often leave spaces between circular plugs of hair. This procedure is very time-consuming and may involve several operations for one transplant, however. The cost can be as much as £6,000.

Older surgical techniques include:

- **Punch grafting** This involves taking a skin graft, usually from the back of the head, and transferring it, follicles intact, to the bald area where holes have been punched. Cost? Several hundred pounds.
- **Flap grafting** This is even more expensive, as a large patch is moved to the bald area. Cost? Over £1,000.
- **Hair stitching** Artificial fibres are implanted in the scalp, again at cost of over £1,000.

Because she had an isolated patch of thinning hair which seemed to be permanent, Abigail of Surrey decided to undergo a hair transplant in Paris with a surgeon who used the modern micro-graft technique. She was concerned that her thinning hair would be an embarrassment at her son's wedding, and thought that a transplant might be the answer. The result was superb. 'I am pleased with the result,' she says. 'But I was very surprised at how sore my scalp was immediately after the operation. The surgeon had suggested that I might like to see the sights of Paris after the operation, but I felt that I just wanted to go home and go to bed.' The cost was £4,000.

You may decide that something less traumatic than surgery is required. Hair weaving is often advertised by high-street beauty clinics. A small hair piece is matched to the client's hair colour and it is woven very tightly into the existing hair. This can, say dermatologists, sometimes cause traction alopecia.

Meanwhile you wander dejectedly in your town — and what do you see? Tempting advertisements, offers to solve your hair problem . . . but how much will it all cost?

CAROLYN: *'In a year I have paid over £2,500 for treatment, including a hair weave.'*

Carolyn is 23. She lives in a city terrace near the car factories of Coventry. A slim, attractive girl, her hair was a striking bush of dark curls, until a year ago.

When her hair started to fall out, Carolyn was still a student. She is now a social worker.

She then had four bald patches. Her doctor was pessimistic. He told her bluntly that she was likely to go bald. Alopecia areata was, after all, in the family. Her great-grandmother had lost her hair completely. She cried. Her doctor prescribed Valium.

'I didn't want tranquillizers. I had quite a battle to persuade him to refer me to a dermatologist and had to wait six months for an appointment.

'While waiting, I followed up a newspaper ad for a commercial hair clinic. They advised a course of treatment which would help my hair. I signed on for 10 at a cost of £327.75. These were followed by a further 10 at the same price. I had some sort of lotion and massage. This seemed to encourage the hair to grow back in the

patches but it was still falling out in other parts of my scalp.

'So I had another 20 treatments and had spent £1,500 by the time my hospital appointment came around. The dermatologist was no more helpful than my GP had been. He predicted I would lose all my hair.

'He felt I wasn't coping well — I was upset again — and he suggested a counsellor at college. This was a waste of time. He was used to dealing with students' problems over their digs and relationships. He had never come across anything like me. He had never heard of baldness in a woman and I spent the time explaining about it.

'I went back to the clinic, very angry. "I've just been to the dermatologist who says I will still go bald", I told them, "and I've paid you all this money to prevent it." Staff at the clinic offered me a hair weave to cover the big bald patch at the front for £1,500, but I had already spent so much that my father was having to help me. He is retired. How could he afford it? In the end, the clinic agreed to charge me only £500 and throw in 10 more massage treatments as well.'

She was pleased with the result. The hair piece matched her own hair and it meant she did not have to wear a wig. Then came the bad news.

'It wasn't until after the weave had been done that they told me about the upkeep. I would have to attend the clinic regularly to have the weave adjusted to keep up with the growth of my existing hair. The cost mounts up. It is working out at around £50 a month.'

Why did it cost so much and why wasn't she told that she would have to go on paying out for its upkeep afterwards?

The branch manager at the hair clinic in Coventry was at pains to explain that Carolyn had been informed: 'We explained that to her before it was fitted.' But Carolyn says she was given no idea of the continual payments involved.

The clinic management proudly flourished a letter written by

Carolyn, thanking them for the treatment and saying how much she liked the weave. Says Carolyn: 'I wrote them a letter of thanks because they asked me to write it. They said that they would be in the running for a case of champagne if their branch got the highest number of letters of appreciation. It was true. I did like the weave. I just didn't like having to pay £2,500 for it. And I am still paying.'

9

HAIR LOSS AND YOUR DIET

There is no doubt that our food really does help – or hinder – hair growth. We have all heard the wise words of the experts: A good diet is essential for healthy hair. 'Of course; we cry. 'Absolutely right! But isn't life bad enough when we are losing our hair, without having to suffer a "sensible" diet!' So we reach for the chocolates . . . the biscuits . . . the double cream . . .

Let's face it, we all know perfectly well that a sensible diet in which we cut out fats and sugar in favour of fibre, fruit, lean meat and fish is an excellent idea. Putting it into practice is a different matter.

The 'comfort eating' syndrome works roughly like this: We are unhappy about our hair loss, self-conscious, embarrassed and gloomy – so that social occasions which were once fun become much more of an effort. Before leaving home we inspect ourselves so often in the mirror that getting ready turns into a nightmare. We make ourselves late. In the end it is hardly worth setting out. We start to dread going out at all and begin to loathe appearing in public, avoiding even our closest friends. We go to amazing lengths – even shopping in supermarkets miles away, far off our usual beat.

At its worst we refuse all invitations and soon, inevitably, we are stuck with long evenings at home, where, bored with finding little chores to do and sick of television, we eventually end up in the kitchen, hovering dangerously near the refrigerator.

Comfort eating happens so easily. Finishing up the scraps in the refrigerator may seem harmless enough – until we realize that one portion of rich rice pudding counts for 1,325 calories! So very soon we are not only hairless but have taken on a distinctly Billy Bunterish look as well.

Why is a sensible diet so important for hair health?

If we are run down and have not been eating properly, the first give-away is our hair, which soon becomes dry, lifeless and dull. But a good eating plan, which includes a balanced amount of protein, vitamins and minerals makes all the difference.

A word of warning: No slimming in a drastic, irresponsible way! Female victims of the slimmers' disease anorexia nervosa who slim right down to the bone and become grotesquely underweight often find that menstruation ceases and they lose hair as well.

For your hair's sake, *eat* – but make it fresh, wholesome food, not over-processed junk. Chemicals, preservation techniques and fertilizers have often damaged these 'foods'. Often the vital minerals and vitamins in foods have been destroyed by other factors as well. Chlorine in drinking water, for instance, can destroy vital vitamin E. Atmospheric pollution, including cigarette smoke, destroys vitamins A and C. Alcohol and the drugs in sleeping tablets can wreck B-complex vitamins.

Vital vitamins for hair growth

Vitamin A (retinol)

Vitamin A helps to maintain the health and growth of hair and skin. A deficiency of vitamin A can sometimes cause follicular hyperkeratosis. This is a condition in which the entire hair follicle is raised by a plug of horny keratin, the protective layer of the skin and nails. Retinoic acid, which is derived from retinol, is sometimes prescribed by dermatologists topically (i.e. applied to the scalp) in the hope of promoting hair growth. Used this way it has been known to help acne or other dry skin conditions. A deficiency can sometimes lead to eyesight problems. Make sure you have your vitamin A; it is found in: kidneys, milk, butter, margarine (this is fortified with vitamin A) spinach, cabbage, carrots (the 'see in the dark' vegetable!), egg yolk and liver.

One cautionary note: A massive overdose of vitamin A can be dangerous as it is a fat-soluble vitamin, i.e. it is stored in the body. A vitamin A overdose can cause headaches, malaise, dryness of the skin and even loss of body hair. If you have any doubts, and particularly if you are pregnant, it is advisable to consult your doctor before you start taking it. (See chart on page 169 for correct nutritional intake.)

B-complex vitamins

These are most important in hair growth and are also thought to improve hair colour. These vitamins can be affected and harmed by such factors as stress, eating too much sugar and an iron deficiency. The B vitamins include the vital folic acid which is so important in pregnancy – and B_{12}, important for mental functions. B_6 (pyridoxine) is vital in the metabolism of protein and amino-acids and particularly helpful to women on HRT, pregnant women and those taking an oral contraceptive.

B-group vitamins are found in soya beans, dairy products, fish, eggs, liver and brewers' yeast.

Vitamin C

Vitamin C is vital for improving the texture of hair. It is biologically active in the production of collagen, the supportive tissue of the skin. As the body cannot store it, a daily intake is essential. This comes from citrus fruit, green vegetables, apples, potatoes, tomatoes, blackcurrants and strawberries.

Vitamin E

Vitamin E is especially important for the hair. It is actually fed to some animals to ensure they grow thick fur. On a cautionary note: No one who is taking anti-coagulant agents for conditions such as thrombosis should take vitamin E without first checking with their doctor. Vitamin E is contained in most vegetable oils, soya, lettuce, nuts, seeds and dairy products; a small amount is found in animal produce.

Vitamin F

Vitamin F keeps the sebaceous glands in good condition and is very important for a healthy scalp and hair growth. Brittle hair, nails and dandruff can be the result of a deficiency of vitamin F. It comes in whole grains, soya, peanuts and wheatgerm.

Important minerals for the hair

Some minerals are just as important as vitamins to the hair.

Iron

Iron is a part of the proteins haemoglobin and myoglobin

which act as oxygen transporters in muscles and red blood cells. Iron deficiency can cause anaemia, with resultant listlessness, fatigue and hair loss.

The best sources of iron are red meat, liver, kidney and heart, parsley, shellfish, egg yolk and cocoa. The iron in green vegetables is often reduced by overcooking.

The hair can also be directly affected by *zinc, selenium, sulphur* and *silicon*. Lack of zinc can also cause miscarriages, stunted growth, rough skin and generally poor health. If zinc is taken in adequate quantities it can improve the condition and growth of the hair as well as being good for the skin, reducing greasiness. Zinc is found in prawns, herrings, meat, nuts, peas and whole grains.

Many hair loss patients have been prescribed a zinc supplement, but sometimes this can cause nausea. Never take it on an empty stomach.

Selenium can help in cases of dandruff. It is an antioxidant which protects the cells of our bodies against the destructive effects of exposure to oxygen. Selenium is found in grains, fish and most whole-foods.

Sulphur is known as the beauty mineral because it is concentrated in hair, nails and skin. It improves the sheen and texture of the hair and is often prescribed for skin complaints such as psoriasis, eczema and dermatitis. It is contained in proteins such as fish, meat, nuts and eggs as well as in green vegetables and onions.

Silicon is found in hair, nails, muscles, skin, teeth and cell walls. If you are deficient in silicon the symptoms are tiredness and dull eyes. Cereal grains are good source of silicon. Silicic acid is absorbed readily from foods and beverages. Also essential for healthy hair are *calcium, magnesium, potassium, phosphorus* and *iodine*.

Are you getting enough?

Faced with the wide list of nutrients we have just considered, you may find yourself wondering whether you are getting the correct amounts in your diet or whether you need to supplement it with health food additives.

As a guide, the Department of Health/UK published in 1979 Recommended Daily Amounts of food, energy and nutrients (RDA). But because this often led to misinterpretation, this guide was in 1991 replaced by the Reference Nutrient Intake – Dietary Reference Values for Food, Energy and Nutrients in the UK. The word 'Recommended' is no longer used, as it led many to believe that it represented the minimum desirable intake for healthy life. In fact, for the majority of the population, the RNI or RDA is substantially more than is needed. The RNI represents the best estimate of those few members of the community with particularly high needs – so if you think the culprit for your hair loss might be your poor diet, the amounts of nutrients in your diet could be worth checking.

Reference Nutrient Intake – The amount of the nutrient that is enough, or more than enough, for 97 per cent of people in a group. If the average intake of a group is at RNI, the risk of deficiency in the group is very small.

Vitamin A. RNI: 700 micrograms (mcg – one millionth of one gram) for an adult male, 600 mcg adult female.

As an overdose of vitamin A can cause liver and bone damage, hair loss, headaches and vomiting, it is important not to take more than 7,500 mcg (women) or 9,000 mcg (men) as a regular intake. A single dose of 300 milligrams (mg) in adults and (100 mg in children) is harmful.

Reference Nutrient Intake for other vitamins (Daily):

Vitamin complex	Adult men	Adult women
Thiamin	.9mg	0.8mg
Riboflavin	1.3mg	1.1mg
Niacin	17mg	13mg
Vitamin B₆	1.4mg	1.2mg
Vitamin B₁₂	1.5mcg	1.5mcg
Folate	200mcg	200mcg
Vitamin C	40mg	40mg*
Vitamin E	4mg	3mg

* (80mg in the case of smokers)

Reference Nutrient Intake for minerals (Daily):

Mineral	Adult men	Adult women
Iron	8.7mg	14.8mg (women with high menstrual losses need more)
Zinc	9.5mg	7.0mg (50mg daily is helpful for those with thin hair)
Selenium	75mcg	60mcg
Sulphur	Below 0.7mg	Below 0.7mg
Silicon	Human requirements are not known. Average UK diet provides 1.2g daily.	
Calcium	700mg	700mg
Magnesium	300mg	270mg
Potassium	3,500mg	3,500mg
Phosphorus	550mg	550mg
Iodine	140mcg	140mcg

Reference Nutrient Intake may seem to suggest very low levels of nutrients, and many people still safely take much higher amounts as a supplement to their diet. Vitamin C, for instance, is taken by many at a level of 500mg daily.

A last word

Help for your hair starts in the kitchen. Whatever you do, please do not overcook vegetables as you are destroying vital vitamins. Avoid too much salt as this causes body tissues to retain water in the scalp tissues.

As a general rule, it should be fairly simple to adjust your diet to include generous helpings of the important vitamins and minerals. A supplement may also be a good plan, plus some brewer's yeast tablets.

> *On the menu*: YOUR HAIR! Grapefruit Cocktail
> Trout with almonds
> Spinach, new potatoes,
> mixed salad
> Baked bananas

Your Eating for Hair Policy
- *Eat*: Low-fat cheese, fish, poultry, red meat, offal, eggs, yogurt, brown rice, nuts, fresh fruit and vegetables, green salads, wholemeal bread and cereal. *Drink*: skimmed milk and plenty of water.
- *Avoid*: Ice-cream, pastries and cakes, salt, junk food, sugar, animal fats, butter, cream, high-fat cheese, white bread and flour, fried and processed foods, chocolate and whole milk.

10

ARE YOU SURE YOU HAVE ALOPECIA?

*'I'm at the end of my tether trying to find support and a
cure for this condition which I have suffered from
for 13 years.'*

FRANCES: *'I feel so guilty when a hairdresser struggles to cover up
a bald patch. He sympathizes, thinking I'm a victim of alopecia. I
can't admit to him that I pull out my hair myself.'*

Frances at 26 is slim, serious and sensitive. Since the age of 12
she has had bald patches in an otherwise normal head of hair. They
are unnoticeable unless she deliberately pulls back the surrounding
hair which camouflages it.

Her problem? Trichotillomania, a nervous stress-related condition
in which victims pull compulsively at their own hair. It is often seen
in young children, rather like a thumb-sucking habit, or in teenage
girls. It often happens in young women of very high intelligence.
Psychiatrists have suggested that it is linked with emotional depriva-
tion in the maternal relationship, or it may be caused by repressed
aggression. Doctors and parents may urge them to stop, but it is a
compulsion. Psychologically, they can't.

As a child, Frances suffered from head lice. *'My scalp would itch
and I would scratch it and start pulling at my hair: single strands,
dragging them out from the crown until I had a bare patch. I used to
pretend to my friends that it had just fallen out.'*

Sometimes patients with this condition refuse to admit it to their *doctors and it can be confused with alopecia, but Frances told her family doctor what was happening. 'My mother took me to see him. He was kind but a bit baffled. He tried to talk with me but it wasn't much help.'*

The habit began at a time when her parents' marriage was under stress. 'They were not quarrelling. No rows, just a quiet, sad home. My father, older than my mother, didn't really know how to play with a child. They both had careers. My father is a teacher, my mother a brilliant mathematician.'

Her hair-pulling habit continued spasmodically through college, where she went to see the students' psychotherapist, 'but it didn't help a lot. I was at war with myself, like being mesmerized. I would pull at it at odd times, then "come to" and find I could see a bare patch.

'I would feel really terrible, knowing it would take months to grow in again. You store up months of trouble for yourself and a vicious circle builds up. Breaking out of the circle is the hardest part.

'The guilt for the damage you've done becomes a source of stress in its own right. And all the time you're trying to pretend to the world that nothing is wrong. You just wish you could hide your head in the sand for three months!'

She has now been working in London for six years and is married. 'The condition came on again with the stress of moving house and coping with a job. My husband didn't notice at all until, on a picnic, I bent my head to look at the dandelions.'

When she first contacted me Frances was upset. 'I'm at the end of my tether trying to find support and a cure for this condition which I have suffered from for 13 years. Why don't people realize that this is as much a worry as having alopecia?' But now, over a year later, she feels she has conquered it. 'I haven't had a bald patch for a year. My hair has all grown in again. This time, I got some counselling and, with a lot of gritting my teeth and a good long holiday in the sun, I think I've done the trick.'

Her days of guilt and struggling to hide the damage with an eyebrow pencil are over, she feels. 'It is in the past. It can be overcome. Although my condition is similar to alopecia in the end result — bald patches — it is really much more like anorexia nervosa or bulimia because it is self-induced and self-destructive. The feelings are those of shame and self-blame. This is very different from being the innocent victim of a medical condition.

'My fantasy is to find a hairdresser who is also a counsellor. People should definitely seek professional help as the condition can mess up your life. It becomes a block preventing you from enjoying anything.'

Trichotillomania, which is more common in females than in males, usually starts either in childhood or the teens. Counselling helps in some cases but a severe case can go on for years. Some women actually pluck out whole heads of hair.

Are you sure you are losing your hair? Or are your eyes deceiving you?

'The woman in my clinic is fiftyish, middle class, well dressed. She has in tow her husband and a photograph album — both to provide evidence that she is in fact losing her hair. She is not. She can't see herself as others see her. She just *thinks* she is going bald.'

Consultant dermatologist Dr Rodney Dawber knows about alopecia. He also knows when the woman complaining of hair loss is suffering from the condition called dysmorphophobia. When she looks in the mirror she sees a distorted image of herself. She has a morbid conviction that she is losing her hair.

'There are a thousand and one reasons why she has this deep-seated conviction that she is balding. She may be suffering from anxiety or depression. She may have difficulties in her relationship with her husband. She may be trying unconsciously to draw attention to herself. She has fixed on this one attribute, her hair, and is probably unconsciously relieved that she has found something to blame.

'My skill as a doctor is to find out what is really wrong. In a skin clinic, a case of dysmorphophobia takes far longer to see than a case of skin cancer. After all, a skin cancer is comparatively straightforward. You know what you are going to do and the patient will comply with what you suggest. It can be dealt with simply. But the danger with a dysmorphophobic patient is that she may attempt suicide. I'm going to have to spend a lot of time with her because she is completely sure she has a scalp disease. She may appear in my clinic outwardly calm and confident. My job is to dig beneath that confidence and find out what's really causing it all.'

Out of the thousands of people for whom alopecia is a fact, there are a few rare cases like this. A woman with a bald head may envy the patient whose hair loss is purely a delusion. 'I wish *I* was just imagining it!' she may sigh.

Dr J. A. Cotterill, consultant dermatologist at Leeds General Infirmary, has studied this condition, which has been described as a 'dermatological non-disease'.[34] He says that it is a 'common and potentially fatal disturbance of cutaneous body image'. He describes it as a symptom of psychiatric disturbance and depression which is often presented to the dermatologist.[35] 'Patients have a disturbance of self-perception which can involve the scalp and the face. Sometimes their disturbance centres not on the scalp, but the breasts in women and the genital area in men.'

Sometimes a woman who has convinced herself that she is

balding, when she definitely is *not*, manages to persuade her husband that it is true and they become involved in what the doctors call a *folie à deux* situation, a joint delusion. Some of these patients, says Dr Cotterill, need their symptoms to avoid situations in their lives which might be painful. They tend to be isolated and to use the condition – their imagined loss of hair – as an excuse to avoid meeting people.

He described the following cases where patients were suffering from dysmorphophobia:

- A secretary, aged 38. Her husband was often away. She had problems at work, as her employer had cancer. She was depressed, tearful and complained that her hair was 'coming out in handfuls'. She was wrong – her hair was not falling out.
- A businessman and director of a company, aged 46, reported a 10-month history of hair loss. Again there was no abnormality.
- An accountant, aged 26, reckoned his hair loss was ruining his life and wrecking his chances with women. The doctors diagnosed: 'an anxious, obsessional personality'. His hair was perfectly normal.

Doctors have suggested that these patients should always be questioned for symptoms of marital difficulties or depression. Dr Cotterill points out that it is not always a good idea to send them to a psychiatrist, as they have mostly made up their own minds which specialist they wish to consult, i.e. the dermatologist.

11

THE FUTURE: WHAT HOPE IS THERE?

*'But isn't there any research going on?
What hope is there of finding a cure?'*

The woman on the phone to Hairline International wants an answer *now*, a magic medicine to drink or a lotion to splash on her scalp to give her what she wants most in the world – a new head of hair. It may sound unlikely but her solution may lie with two humble creatures she would evict on sight from her sitting room: the rat and the mouse.

In Britain, scientists at Dundee University have been working for over 20 years with cells at the base of the hair follicle, called the dermal papillae, which seem to control the production of hair. They have been using papilla cells taken from rats as human cells are in many ways similar to those of the rat. A multi-national industry has donated a million pounds to this research.

Meanwhile, in Sheffield, consultant dermatologist Dr Andrew Messenger has found a method of culturing dermal papilla cells from human follicles.[36] It is an incredibly fiddly job, he explains, 'but, once this is achieved, cell cultures can be established.' He hopes this will be the breakthrough – the key to solving many problems in growing hair.

These techniques will allow the use of wider methods for

studying reactions in alopecia, the action of hormones on hair growth and the effect of drugs. It may be possible to use dermal papilla cells or their products directly as a form of treatment.

In Salt Lake City, Utah, dermatologists have been experimenting with scalp grafts from people who have lost their hair.[37] These are grafted on to nude mice. The researchers use these animals because they are unable to mount a rejection response. If they grafted human skin on to any other type of mouse it would be rapidly rejected. The researchers wanted an answer to the question: Is the disease alopecia areata inherent to affected tissue or secondary to circulating factors?

As a result hair grew on the nude mice. This proved that hairgrowth ability is normal in alopecia/areata/totalis/universalis. The factors causing it are circulating in the bloodstream. When the hair follicles are removed from these factors by being transplanted, the hair is able to grow.

The nude mice were also treated with cyclosporine, the immuno-suppressive drug used in the treatment of transplant patients. Cyclosporine was known to cause excessive hair growth as a side-effect (see page 156). In this research, the cyclosporine affected hair growth to the extent that, by day 78, the number of hairs per graft and the mean length of the hair had increased significantly over untreated groups.

Research was also carried out at Wayne State University, Detroit, on diazoxide, a drug used to treat low blood sugar. Like minoxidil, it has been found to encourage hair growth as a side-effect.

At New York University, researchers have tried to discover the triggers which turn the hair growth phase – anagen – into the resting – telogen – phase. For years, research has centred on the lymphocytes, the cells which apparently initiate the immune response and the destructive process. The lymphocytes which trigger the immune response are thought to be the helper T lymphocytes. Suppressor T lymphocytes, which turn off the immune response and so end the destructive process, are very much in the minority in areas of alopecia areata.

Says Dr Messenger: 'Suppressor T lymphocytes are present in the cellular infiltrate in and around hair follicles in alopecia areata. But helper T lymphocytes predominate. The helper/suppressor T cell ratio tends to be similar in most inflammatory diseases – not just AA – being around three or four to one.'

Dr Brian Jegasothy, Professor of Dermatology at the University of Pennsylvania, has found in research that the suppressor T lymphocytes are so much in the minority that they are almost absent among the cells in the area of alopecia.[38] 'Concerning treatment', says Professor Jegasothy, 'it might be desirable to reduce helper T cell activity specifically or increase suppressor T cell activity in areas of hair loss, but this approach is not possible using currently available treatments.'

Professor Jegasothy has found that another cell, the Langerhans cell, is increased by as much as 10 times in alopecia areata. These cells appear to change foreign material into a form which initiates the immunological process. The most exciting aspect of these findings is that Langerhans cells can be decreased or eliminated by local treatment with PUVA.' He used PUVA (see page 155) applying psoralens topically – to the skin – with eight patients who had total hair loss. They all grew terminal (normal) hair.

'I'd pay anything to get my hair back'

All this research, fascinating though it is, is still offering hope to alopecia sufferers *only* in the long term, when they want their hair back *now*.

One of the most disturbing things about the lack of structured health help is that many people are prepared to raise enormous sums for private medicine in the hope of getting their hair back. They head for London's Harley Street, full of hope and clutching a cheque book. A doctor in the private sector can look them straight in the eye and ask for a four-figure sum for his treatment . . . which won't be coming from balding millionaires or millionairesses, but from ordinary people desperate for medical help for their problem. They will raise the money if they can, to the advantage of the private practitioner, even though both doctor and patient know there is no guarantee that hair will return.

JANE, 47, said: 'I thought that if I went to Harley Street I was paying for the best treatment. I'd been told I had male pattern baldness and thought an endocrinologist would help. His treatment was intensive — at least he found out that I was deficient in oestrogen. But it went on for two years and by the time it finished I had spent over £2,000. I still haven't got my hair back. He did warn me at the beginning that it might not work, so I suppose it was fair enough. But it did cost a lot of money. People should realize that if they have private treatment, it will be very expensive.'

'How do I know what type of hair loss I have?

The worst thing about losing your hair is often doing the dreary round of doctors, trying to find the right specialist. No doctor seems to consider the whole patient or really investigate the cause. Dermatologists fight shy of any question about hormones and it is unlikely that a woman will see an endocrinologist at all, unless there is evidence of virilization, menstrual or infertility problems. Surely this situation is highly unsatisfactory from the patient's point of view?

'Yes', said one consultant endocrinologist, Dr Christopher H. Mortimer. 'I want to co-ordinate the specialties so that we can assess – in one clinic – the cause of the hair loss and the complete hormonal and medical condition of the patient.'

Seeing himself as a pioneer, Dr Mortimer founded the Endocrine and Dermatology Centre, a £1.5 million project in London's Harley Street, based in a listed building which had been expensively equipped and renovated. Formerly a research lecturer in medicine with the Medical Research Council at St Bartholomew's Hospital, London, he developed techniques for the measurement and clinical application of the brain hormones which control fertility and body growth. He also carried out research into the hormones which cause and protect against common baldness in both sexes.

'My aim is to provide an internationally co-ordinated network so that patients who have lost their hair can be referred here for treatment. I have on my staff a nucleus of highly trained endocrinologists with extensive research experience both in this country and the United States. A reverse brain drain!*

'When a patient comes to us we build up a complete picture. In a woman, we ask: Is she on the pill? It's been known for years that some of the progestogens in the pill can actually precipitate androgen – male hormone – based conditions such as acne vulgaris, hirsuties or scalp hair loss. After a long talk, I send her home. I ask her to think and work out answers to the following questions: What is her

* Sadly, Dr Mortimer died suddenly in 1991. Nevertheless his work is being continued by Dr Wayne Perry, MB, Ch B., MRCP, at the Endocrine Centre, 69 Wimpole Street, London W1M 7DE.

opinion of me? Can I help her or not? Has she really got a problem? Am I bonkers? Or is there hope?

'When she is certain she trusts me, she can come back. On day 21 of her cycle, we will obtain a full endocrine profile with blood and urine tests, check on her physical health, including heart, gynaecological history and general medical condition. We will make certain there is no evidence of tumours, diabetes or anaemia. Clinical photography follows and a hair density study which may include a scalp biopsy'. This is where a tiny piece of tissue is taken from the scalp for study under the microscope.

Dr Mortimer went on to complete research studies on hair density. 'It is clearly pointless to get involved in hair loss problems without first checking the patient's hair density against that of a normal individual.'

Further tests were carried out on the patient and a record kept of his or her response at three, six, nine and twelve months. 'It's a full year of treatment and assessment but by the end of it we have a full picture and the basis for future medical management.'

Dr Mortimer's experience included detailed research into the treatment of women aged from 17 to 60 using anti-androgen therapy. An increase in hair density was achieved in each of the patients in the original study with a similar pattern of response in wider trials.[39]

He used various treatments and favoured the use of diphencyprone (see page 151).

Dr Mortimer saw a close relationship between endocrine and dermatology conditions. The centre will integrate the various medical disciplines to provide a greater understanding of hair abnormalities.

'More attention should be paid to the psychological damage to a woman when she loses her hair. Balding is often an acceptable – if undesirable – condition in a man beyond a certain age, but even minimal scalp hair loss at any time generates considerable anxiety in women. If it becomes clinically obvious, severe psychological symptoms may occur, with feelings of loss of femininity and self-confidence. One of our patients had severe depression after two years of hair loss. This resolved completely during anti-androgen therapy without the need for psychotropic drugs.'

The problem with Dr Mortimer's plan is the cost. He once estimated that the cost to the patient would be around £3,500 during the first year, which would probably include systemic cyclical anti-androgen therapy, prescribed as capsules by mouth. The high cost would obviously put it out of the range of most people, unless private medical insurance companies were prepared to help. This is unlikely, although one firm has agreed to reimburse those insured with it for at least a part of the treatment.

'My hope is to find a means for funding patients myself – possibly through the large pharmaceutical companies involved in my research. A breakthrough in cost will happen when topical anti-androgen therapy becomes available for routine use.' The hope is that this will be less expensive than the capsules. It will be a lotion applied to the scalp.

'There is so much to be done in this field: tissue cultures, new drug treatments, hair follicle cloning – even individual fibre replacement! It may sound like science fiction but the era of endodermal research has only just begun and anything is possible.'

12

WHEN HAIR GROWS BACK

'Sometimes — just sometimes — there is good news.'

Sometimes the hair grows back of its own accord. About one-third of all cases recover after the first episode of alopecia areata — and never get another bald patch. Two-thirds get a relapse within six months but there is still a good chance that their condition will clear up ultimately.

TRACEY is 24, an ambitious, outgoing girl with a thriving career as promotions manager of a jewellery company.

At 10, she lost all her hair. She also suffers from eczema and asthma — both conditions run in her family — so the prognosis was not good and her consultant took her parents aside to warn them that her hair would probably never return.

Tracey's parents both had careers. Her mother is a musician, her father is in market research. 'They were very good. So was my sister. The whole family spoiled me. My parents were worried sick about it, wondering what they had done wrong.'

But being bald throughout secondary school changed her, she thinks. 'I deliberately made myself inconspicuous. I would not do anything which drew attention to myself. I felt I looked hideous — well, not hideous exactly, more like an alien from another planet! Grown-ups would make remarks, ask whether I was wearing a wig. I just went quiet, embarrassed, and couldn't answer. There were things at school I couldn't do and I never understood why the teachers were so insistent that I do them. They knew I had to wear a wig. Why did they make me do the high jump, when it would almost certainly fall off? People were insensitive and I didn't want to talk about it. All through childhood, I remember the subject being very hush-hush. My parents didn't mention it. After all, it was a condition no one knew much about. You just had to get on with it. One teacher ordered me to wash my face — I was only wearing make-up to match in with the wig. I was so hurt, but she said I looked "painted".

'I was constantly worried and unsure of myself. I thought the wigs looked all right at the time but, looking back, I can see that people could tell a mile off. Some people are so bloody rude, the ones you come across daily in shops and so on. I didn't want attention. But I still had a good social life. I used to work at a local disco on Saturdays and get to know boys. At 17, though, I hadn't any boy-friends. I think the opportunity was there but I was very cool about it. I suppose I just didn't want to get involved in case they had to see me without my wig. I was just "holding back" all the time, never being completely myself.'

Then suddenly . . . the good news!

'I had always believed my hair would grow back and after four or five years I started to notice the odd tuft, the odd eyelash. I realized that it was slowly growing again. Soon it all came back. It was the same mid-brown colour and it covered my head all over. We were going on a family holiday which was good because it covered the break between a wig and my own hair again. I felt marvellous and my relationships with boys just took off after that!'

But at 22, her hair started falling out again. *'I was really shat-tered, sobbing all over doctors, really down and despairing. Patches came and went. I started to will my hair not to fall out. I would lie* on my bed and command the hair roots to stay in place! At this stage I had to tell my lover about my hair history. I had never mentioned it before. Oddly enough, he was all right. He seemed understanding about the bald patches but I was aware that he had never seen me totally hairless. I'm not sure that he would have coped if the whole lot had fallen out.

'Luckily it hasn't come to that. My father paid for me to go to a dermatologist privately and he gave me injections into my scalp which seemed to help. I also believe in yoga and the power of the mind. I've recently taken a big new job in marketing and I'm just going to believe that it will never happen again — perhaps the odd patch, but nothing like what I went through before.'

Tracey's good news is not unusual. Sometimes hair regrows. A woman wrote to me from Regent's Park, London, about her daughter, aged 23. 'Her lovely blonde hair came out at an alarming rate over a period of about a month. At an age when one is looking for a marriage partner, she found herself too tense and upset to form any relationships.

'Now, nearly four years later, her hair has grown, long and thick enough for her to stop wearing a wig. The hair is dark not fair and she still has only a few eyelashes. However, we are thankful that her hair has recovered and — hopefully — that this is the end of a very traumatic experience.'

Her hair regrew without medical treatment, a classic case reinforcing the view of the doctor who says: 'Leave it alone. It will come back by itself.' But it also happens after weeks of painstaking effort by a dermatologist, as in Emma Jane's case.

EMMA JANE had tried for years to get her hair back but it remained so patchy that she was forced to wear a wig. For years she had done nothing on the advice of doctors, then she was lucky enough to find a dermatologist who tried various topical prepara-

tions. 'Suddenly', says Emma Jane, 'my hair just grew! I walked into my dermatologist's surgery without a wig. He looked up and grinned. "Great," he said. And for the first time in years I don't have to wear wigs.'

The hopeful thing about alopecia areata is that the hair follicles do not seem to be destroyed by the disease. When people who have been without hair for five, ten, even forty years, say 'I live in hope' they are not wearing rose-tinted spectacles. Hair recently returned to a woman in Leeds who had been without it for 54 years. It can come back at *any* time. All it needs is that mysterious trigger to set it off.

So *never* give up hope.

POSTSCRIPT

'But I am losing my hair now.
Where do I go for help?'

When it happened to me, I could find nowhere, which is why I founded Hairline as a national support network for women who have lost or are losing their hair. We soon had to enrol male patients who convinced us that they suffered with alopecia areata as much as women. We also enrolled the parents of children with hair loss. Soon we had members all over the UK, Europe and the Far East.

In the USA, action similar to mine was being taken by Ashley Siegel, herself an AA victim. She advertised for other sufferers to contact her. Their organization – the National Alopecia Areata Foundation – now stretches from coast to coast and in the last six years has raised $600 million for medical research into alopecia.

I realized quickly how important hair loss can become to the individual. I was horrified when one girl told me: 'I would rather have had thalidomide and been born without arms, than to have lost my hair.' I was angry with her at the time, it seemed such a wicked thing to say. But I realized she meant it. I also understood when people told me: 'I would rather have asthma – or appendicitis – or pneumonia.' Perhaps this is because these are 'normal' everyday conditions. They do not carry the stigma or the humiliation of losing your hair, or wreak such havoc with your looks. There are also conventional paths to treatment, not the bewildering battle to find a doctor prepared to help.

'So what happened in your case? Did you get your hair back?'

Everyone asks me that question. After 11, nearly 12 years, I can reply, at last, after years in wigs and headscarves, YES, MY HAIR HAS REGROWN. I now have long dark hair again. Because of the eccentric nature of this condition, I cannot be 100 per cent certain that it regrew because of the modern medical treatment I had. I was prescribed topical minoxidil (Regaine) and I am 90 per cent certain that it helped.

In the end, I have been lucky. I have people to thank: my parents, for never making it a 'big deal' and behaving as though it was as normal as catching flu; my husband, who did a great job of 'not noticing' even in the early days when I looked more like an extra-terrestrial than a wife; and my 12-year-old daughter, Kathryn, who at the age of six put the whole thing into perspective. I had been a little concerned in case 'My mummy wears a wig' found its way into her school diary, so I had prepared my story. 'You see', I said, over a cup of tea, 'after you were born I had a skin disease and all my hair fell out. It happens to quite a lot of people. So I've had to wear a wig.' Kathryn was silent, digesting this – I thought. I waited for some profound follow-up question. She opened her mouth. 'Please may I have another lollipop?' she asked, and never mentioned my hair again!

I also thank the brave members of Hairline, who backed

me through the slogging days of asking questions, trying to find out all I could about hair loss and what could be done about it, generally pestering people, I suppose. It has been these wonderful people who have been brave enough to congratulate me on my new head of hair. I had thought that perhaps they might be upset, particularly if mine had regrown and theirs had not. Imagine my delight then, that they have all, without exception, been pleased for me and told me 'It gives us hope.'

I have to thank Dr David Fenton, the dermatologist who enthusiastically runs the Hair and Nail Unit at St Thomas's Hospital, London. He never tired of varying his treatment in the long struggle to provoke my lazy hair into growing again. I was lucky to find him. Such men are rare.

I was also fortunate to have been a journalist, often writing on medical and sociological subjects, so I was accustomed to knocking on doors and asking questions. I was able to find the experts who would help me.

The people who suffer most from severe hair loss are the ones who take a doctor's word for it that nothing can be done – as I did at the beginning, who cry over the Hairline phone: 'It took me four appointments to persuade my GP to send me to a dermatologist – and then there was no treatment he could offer!'

These patients are not neurotics, imagining that a few lost hairs are a crisis. They are people who have suddenly lost *all* or nearly all their hair. Too often, the effect on their lives is underestimated.

As one courageous woman of 65 told me: 'To start losing one's hair as a teenager and to see it getting worse is extremely demoralizing. I have never had a normal head of hair. I have always "put on an act" and assumed a cheerfulness and contentment with life but have suffered privately from awful depression and feelings of hopelessness. It has always seemed to me that nothing has been done for women like us, as ours is not a physically disabling handicap. But emotionally it greatly diminishes the quality of one's life. So much money, research and medical help is devoted to self-inflicted ailments these days but very little, it seems, is devoted to our problem. Perhaps because we are too ashamed to talk about it.'

It doesn't hurt. It is not life-threatening. But sudden hair loss can make a fair old mess of your life if you let it.

You are not going to let it. If you have followed my survival plan, you will work at it, batter down doors to find experts who will help, and buy the wigs and accessories which arm you for the fight to look good again, to throw off the feeling of being a 'freak' and claw your way back in to the human race.

I promise that you will look good, perhaps even better than you ever looked before.

You are going to survive alopecia.

Aren't you?

REFERENCES

1 Drs M. B. Sulzberger, V. H. Witten and A. W. Kopf, 'Diffuse Alopecia in Women', *Archives of Dermatology* (1960), 81:556.

2 Dr F. E. Cormia, 'Alopecia from Oral Contraceptives', *Journal of the American Medical Association* (1967), 201:635.

3 Drs Arthur Rook and Rodney Dawber, *Diseases of the Hair and Scalp*, (Blackwell Scientific, 1982).

4 Drs E. Panconesi and G. Mantellassi, *Rassegna di Dematologia e Sifilografia* (1955), 8:121.

5 Dr I. Macalpine, 'Is Alopecia Areata Psychosomatic?', *British Journal of Dermatology* (1958), 70:117.

6 Dr A. J. M. Penders, 'Alopecia Areata and Atopy', *Dermatologica* (1968) 136:395.

7 Drs S. A. Muller and R. K. Winkelmann, 'Alopecia Areata', *Archives of Dermatology* (1963), 88:290.

8 Dr T. Ikeda, 'A New Classification of Alopecia Areata', *Dermatologica* (1965), 131:421.

9 Drs M. N. El Makhzangy, V. Wynn and Daphne M. Lawrence, *Clinical Endocrinology* (1979), 10:39–45.

10 Dr E. Hoffman, H. G. Meiers and A. Hubbes 'Wirkungen von Antikonzeptiva auf Alopecia Androgenetica, Seborrhea Oleosa, Akne Vulgaria und Hirsutismus', *Deutsche Medizinische Wochenshrift* (1974), 99:2151–7.

11 Professor Vera Price, Department of Dermatology, University of California School of Medicine. International Society of

Tropical Dermatology (1979), vol. 18, no. 2.

12 Dr H. Zaun, Ovulationshemmer in der Dematologia (1972).

13 Dr W. A. D. Griffiths, St John's (now part of St Thomas's Hospital), London. *British Journal of Dermatology* (1973), 88:31.

14 Drs S. A. Walker and S. Rothman, 'Alopecia Areata: A Statistical Study', *Journal of Investigative Dermatology* (1950), 14:403.

15 Dr Sigfrid A. Muller, *Epidemiological Survey* (1950–1974).

16 Drs Sigfrid A. Muller and R. K. Winkelmann, 'Alopecia Areata', *Archives of Dermatology* (1963), 88:290.

17 Drs S. A. Walker and S. Rothman, 'Alopecia Areata: A Statistical Study', *Journal of Investigative Dermatology* (1950), 14:403.

18 Drs Sigfrid A. Muller and R. K. Winkelmann, 'Alopecia Areata', *Archives of Dermatology* (1963), 88:290.

19 Dr C. L. Schmitt, 'Trauma as a Factor in the Production of Alopecia Universalis', *Pennsylvania Medical Journal* (1953), 56:975.

20 Dr T. Ikeda, 'A New Classification of Alopecia Areata', *Dermatologica* (1965), 131:421.

21 Dr A. R. Zappacosta, 'Reversal of Baldness in Patient Receiving Minoxidil for Hypertension', *New England Journal of Medicine* (1980), 303:1480–1.

22 Drs David Fenton and John Wilkinson, *British Medical Journal* (1983), 287:1015–17.

23 Dr Gerda Frentz, *Acta Derm Venereol* (1985), 65:172–5.

24 Drs Clodagh M. King, Brian Harrop, Vinay K. Dave, *British Medical Journal* (1983), 287:1380.

25 Drs S. Lewis Jones and C. F. J. Vickers, *British Medical Journal* (1983), 287:1380.

26 Drs J. M. Maitland, R. D. Aldridge, R. A. Main, M. I. White, A. D. Ormerod, *British Medical Journal* (1984), 288:794.

27 Drs Colin Hindson, Jon Spiro, Ailean Taylor, Eilean Pratt, *British Medical Journal* (1984), 288:1087.

28 Drs V. C. Weiss, D. P. West, C. E. Mueller, 'Topical Minoxidil in Alopecia Areata', *J Am Acad Dermatology* (1981).

29 Drs V. C. Weiss, Dennis P. West, Tony S. Fu, Lisa A. Robinson, Brian Cook, Rhona L. Cohen, Donald L. Chambers, *Arch Dermatol* (1984), 120:457–63.

30 Drs V. C. Fiedler Weiss, Dennis P. West, Cunera M. Buys, Jean A. Rumsfield, *Arch Dermatol* (1986), 122:180–2.

31 Drs Victoria M. Yates, Clodagh M. King, Brian Harrop, *British Medical Journal* (1984), 288:1087.

32 Dr J. A. Savin, *British Medical Journal* (1982), 284:445–6.

33 Drs E. L. Rhodes, W. Dolman, C. Kennedy, R. R. Taylor, 'Alopecia Areata Regrowth Induced by *Primula Obconica*', *British Journal of Dermatology* (1981), 104:339.

34 Dr C. K. Meador, 'The Art and Science of Non-Disease', *New England Journal of Medicine* (1965), 272:92–5.

35 Dr J. A. Cotterill, 'Dermatological Non-Disease: A Common and Potentially Fatal Disturbance of Cutaneous Body Image', *British Journal of Dermatology* (1981), 104:611.

36 Dr A. G. Messenger, *British Journal of Dermatology* (1985), 113:639–40.

37 Drs A. Gilhar and G. G. Krueger, *Arch Dermatol* (1987), 123:44–51.

38 Dr Brian Jegasothy, Professor Dept of Dermatology, University of Pennsylvania, National Alopecia Areata Foundation, 1984.

39 Dr Christopher Mortimer, 'Effective Medical Treatment for Common Baldness in Women', *Clinical and Experimental Dermatology* (1984).

USEFUL ADDRESSES

Hairline International – The Alopecia Patients' Society
Lyons Court
1668 High Street
Knowle, West Midlands
B93 0LY
(Please enclose A4 size SAE.)

or

Wayside House
191 Station Lane
Lapworth
Solihull, West Midlands
B94 6JG
(Please enclose A4 size SAE.)

INDEX